PULMONARY FUNCTION TESTS
A Guide for the Student and House Officer

PULMONARY FUNCTION TESTS
A Guide for the Student and House Officer

Edited by

Albert Miller, M.D.

Clinical Professor of Medicine
Clinical Professor of Community Medicine
Director, Pulmonary Laboratory
Mount Sinai Medical School
New York, New York

Grune & Stratton, Inc.

Harcourt Brace Jovanovich, Publishers

Orlando   New York   San Diego   London
San Francisco   Tokyo   Sydney   Toronto

Library of Congress Cataloging-in-Publication Data

Pulmonary function tests.

Includes bibliographies and index.
1. Pulmonary function tests.   2. Lungs—Diseases
Diagnosis.   I. Miller, Albert.   [DNLM: 1. Respiratory
Function Tests.   WF 141 P98243]
RC734.P84P84135   1987   616.2'4075   86-29418
ISBN 0-8089-1764-1

Grune & Stratton, Inc.
Orlando, FL 32887

Distributed in the United Kingdom by
Grune & Stratton, Ltd.
24/28 Oval Road, London NW 1

Library of Congress Catalog Number 86-29418
International Standard Book Number 0-8089-1764-1

Printed in the United States of America
87 88 89 90   10 9 8 7 6 5 4 3 2 1

CONTENTS

PREFACE

This guide to the use of pulmonary function tests is intended for the student, house officer, or physician interested in how the tests are utilized in clinical respiratory medicine. We shall concern ourselves only with those tests that are helpful in diagnostic and therapeutic decision making: dynamic lung volumes—forced vital capacity (FVC), forced expiratory volume-one second (FEV_1), expiratory and inspiratory flow rates, maximum voluntary ventilation (MVV); full lung volumes—functional residual capacity (FRC), total lung capacity (TLC), and residual volume (RV); diffusing capacity of the lung (D_L), and arterial blood gases. This book does not cover such topics as measurements of mechanical forces, more complicated tests of distribution of ventilation, or neural control mechanisms, since these are of interest primarily to research investigators or specialized centers. Similarly, the many epidemiologic applications of pulmonary function tests are not discussed. Interested readers are referred to our companion volume, *Pulmonary Function Tests in Clinical and Occupational Lung Disease,* for information in these areas.

In order to point out the clinical usefulness of pulmonary function tests, we have defined them and placed them within a pathophysiologic context. In order for him or her to relate a test result to a specific patient, the reader is introduced to prediction equations, and specific recommendations are made concerning which of the many equations to use and how to use them to define "normal values" and degrees of impairment. The various kinds of impairment that are identified by pulmonary function tests are delineated, and the relevance of these physiologic impairments to clinical findings and pathologic alterations is stressed. Case presentations illustrate the uses of the various tests. The last chapters discuss the more specific, but clinically important areas of bronchodilation and bronchoprovoction, pulmonary function testing in children, disability evaluation, respiratory abnormalities during sleep, and ability to withstand surgery.

— ABBREVIATIONS AND TERMINOLOGY —

The terminology and abbreviations of the American College of Chest Physicians/ American Thoracic Society (ACCP/ATS) joint committee have generally been used, following the practice of Clausen in 1982. A dash above any symbol ($\bar{X}$) indicates a mean value; a dot ($\dot{X}$) indicates a rate. In accordance with practice in the United States, traditional units are used instead of Standard International units.

Additional abbreviations (set off by parentheses) are used in this book for convenience. In tribute to long usage, such terms as *MMF* and *PFR* are used interchangeably with $FEF_{25-75\%}$ and $\dot{V}max$, respectively. Similarly, *cc* and *mm Hg* are used interchangeably with *ml* and *Torr*. The FEV_1/FVC ratio is shown as a decimal (eg, 0.75) rather than a percentage (75%) to avoid confusion with FEV_1 as a percentage of predicted. The spectrum of chronic obstructive lung disease is referred to as *CAO* for chronic airways obstruction and that of interstitial lung disease as ILD.

A modification of the guidelines for rounding off values suggested in 1973 by the European Coal and Steel Community is useful:

1. Maximum volumes >2 L are rounded off to the nearest 50 ml, eg, VC recorded as 4.863 L becomes 4.85 L.
2. Maximum volumes <2 L are rounded off to the nearest 10 ml.
3. Tidal volumes, minute volumes, O_2 consumption, and CO_2 production are rounded off to the nearest 10 ml.
4. MVV is rounded off to the nearest liter.

A	Alveolar
a	Arterial
(ACCP)	American College of Chest Physicians
an or anat	Anatomic
(AT)	Anaerobic threshold
ATPD	Ambient temperature and pressure, dry
ATPS	Ambient temperature and pressure, saturated with water vapor at these conditions
(ATS)	American Thoracic Society
aw or AW	Airways
B	Barometric

b	Blood
(BD)	Bronchodilator, bronchodilitation
BTPS	Body temperature, ambient pressure, saturated with water (vapor pressure 47 mm Hg at 37°)
C	A general symbol for compliance, volume change per unit of applied pressure; also, content
c	Capillary
C/v_L	Specific compliance of the lung
(CAO)	Chronic airways obstruction
(CC)	Closing capacity
C_{dyn}	Dynamic compliance, compliance measured at point of zero gas flow at the mouth during active breathing. The respiratory frequency should be designated; eg, $C_{dyn}40$
C_{st}	Static compliance; measurements made during interruption of air flow
(CV)	Closing volume; also coefficient of variation
D	Dead space or wasted ventilation (used as qualifying symbol, eg, V_D)
D	Diffusing capacity
D_k	Diffusion coefficient or permeability constant as described by Krogh: $DL \cdot (P_B - P_{H_2O}/V_A)$
D_m	Diffusing capacity of the alveolar capillary membrane (STPD)
$D_L(CO$ or $O_2)$	Diffusing capacity of the lung expressed as ml (STPD) of gas uptake per mm Hg alveolar-capillary pressure difference per minute. A modifier is used to designate the technique, eg, D_LCO_{SB}, D_LCO_{SS}
D_L/V_A	Diffusion (STPD) per unit of alveolar volume (BTPS)
E	Expired
(ecg)	Electrocardiograph(ic), electrocardiogram
(EPP)	Equal pressure point; see R_{us}
ERV	Expiratory reserve volume; the maximal volume of air exhaled from the resting end-expiratory level
est	Estimated
(ET)	End-tidal
f	Respiratory frequency per minute
F	Fractional concentration of a gas
FEF_{max}	The maximal forced expiratory flow achieved during an FVC (see PFR)
FEF_x	Forced expiratory flow after x portion (in percent or L) of the FVC has been exhaled; eg, $FEF_{75\%}$ is the instantaneous flow after 75% of the FVC has been exhaled. Note difference from volume designated for $\dot{V}_{max}$

$FEF_{25-75\%}$	Mean forced expiratory flow during the middle half of the FVC (formerly called the maximum mid-expiratory flow rate or MMF[R])
$FEF_{200-1200}$	Mean forced expiratory flow between 200 ml and 1200 ml of the FVC (formerly called the maximum expiratory flow rate or MEF[R])
FET_x	The forced expiratory time for a specified portion of the FVC; eg, $FET_{95\%}$ is the time required to deliver the first 95% of the FVC and $FET_{25-75\%}$ is the time required to deliver the $FEF_{25-75\%}$
$FEV_{(t)}$	Forced expiratory volume, (timed). Times (in seconds) are designated by subscripts, eg, $FEV_{0.75}$, FEV_1, etc.
FIF_x	Forced inspiratory flow. As in the case of the FEF, appropriate modifiers are used to designate the volume at which flow is measured.
FRC	Functional residual capacity; the sum of RV and ERV; the volume of air remaining in the lungs at the resting end-expiratory position
(F-V)	Flow-volume (curve)
FVC	Forced vital capacity
G	Conductance, the reciprocal of R
G_{aw}/V_L	Specific conductance, expressed per liter of lung volume at which G is measured (also referred to as SG_{aw})
(HR)	Heart rate
I	Inspired
IC	Inspiratory capacity; the sum of IRV and V_T
(ILD)	Interstitial lung disease
IRV	Inspiratory reserve volume; the maximal volume of air inhaled from the end-inspiratory level
L	Lung
max	Maximal
MBC	Maximum breathing capacity
(MEF[R])	See $FEF_{200-1200}$
MEFV)	Maximum expiratory flow-volume (curve)
(MET)	See $FET_{25-75\%}$
(MMF[R])	See $FET_{25-75\%}$
MVV	Maximal voluntary ventilation. The volume of air expired or inspired during repetitive maximal respiratory effort, expressed in L/min
P	Physiologic; also probability
P	Pressure, blood or gas
(PA)	Pulmonary artery; also posteroanterior

(PC) or (PD)	Provocative concentration or provocative dose; the dose of an agent used in bronchial provocation testing that results in a defined change in a specific physiologic parameter. The parameter tested and the percent change in this parameter are indicated, eg, PD_{20} FEV_1 for a 20% decrease in FEV_1
(PDS)	Physiologic dead space; see V_D
PEF (or PFR)	Peak expiratory flow or peak flow rate, generally measured with a peak flow meter
pl	Pleural
(P max$_E$ or P_E max)	Maximum expiratory pressure at the mouth (measured at or near TLC)
($P_{max/I}$ or P_I max)	Maximum inspiratory pressure at the mouth (measured at or near RV or FRC)
P_{st}	Static transpulmonary pressure at a specific lung volume; eg, P_{st}TLC is static recoil pressure measured at TLC (maximal recoil pressure)
Q	Blood volume
$\dot{Q}$	Blood flow
R	A general symbol for resistance, pressure per unit flow; also, the respiratory exchange ratio in general, $\dot{V}CO_2/\dot{V}O_2$
R_{aw}	Airway resistance
(RB)	Rebreathing
RQ	Respiratory quotient
R_{us}	Resistance of the airways on the alveolar side (*upstream*) of the point (EPP) where intraluminal pressure equals Ppl, measured during maximum expiratory flow
RV	Residual volume; that volume of air remaining in the lungs after maximal exhalation. The method of measurement should be indicated.
S	Saturation
(SA)	Small airway
(SB)	Single breath
(SD)	Standard deviation
(SEE)	Standard error of the estimate
(SS)	Steady state
STPD	Standard conditions; temperature 0°C, pressure 760 mm Hg, and dry (0 water vapor)
t	Time
T	Tidal
TGV	Thoracic gas volume; the volume of gas within the thoracic cage as measured by body plethysmography
(TV)	Tidal volume

UAO	Upper airway obstruction
V	Gas volume. The particular gas as well as its pressure, water vapor, and other special conditions must be specified in text or indicated by appropriate qualifying symbols
$\dot{V}$	Gas volume per unit time, eg, ventilation in L/min; also, rate of gas flow
v	Venous
$\bar{v}$	Mixed venous
$\dot{V}_A$	Alveolar ventilation per minute (BTPS)
V_c	Pulmonary capillary blood (preferably Qc) in intimate association with alveolar gas
VC	Vital capacity
$\dot{V}CO_2$	Carbon dioxide production per minute (STPD)
$\dot{V}_D$	Ventilation per minute of the physiologic dead space (wasted ventilation), BTPS, defined by the following equation: $\dot{V}_D = \dot{V}_E(PaCO_2 - P_ECO_2/PaCO_2 - P_ICO_2)$
V_D	The physiologic dead-space volume defined as $\dot{V}_D/f$
$V_D$an	Volume of the anatomic dead space (BTPS)
$\dot{V}_E$	Expired volume (usually of ventilation (per minute) (BTPS)
$\dot{V}_I$	Inspired volume (usually of ventilation (per minute) (BTPS)
Viso$\dot{V}$	Volume of isoflow; the volume above RV at which the expiratory flow rates become identical when flow—volume loops performed after breathing room air and helium-oxygen mixtures are superimposed
$\dot{V}O_2$	Oxygen consumption per minute (STPD)
$\dot{V}_{max}$	Forced expiratory flow, related to the total lung capacity or the absolute volume of the lung at which the measurement is made. *Modifiers refer to the amount of lung volume remaining when the measurement is made.* For example: $\dot{V}_{max}75\%$ is instantaneous forced expiratory flow when the lung is at 75% of its TLC; $\dot{V}3.0$ is instantaneous forced expiratory flow when the lung volume is 3.0 L. Note difference from volume designated for FEF.
V_T	Tidal volume; TV is also commonly used

Blood-Gas Measurements

Abbreviations for these values are readily composed by combining the general symbols defined above. The following are examples:

$PaCO_2$	Arterial carbon dioxide tension
$C(a-\bar{v})O_2$	Arteriovenous oxygen content difference
CcO_2	Oxygen content of (pulmonary end) capillary blood
F_ECO	Fractional concentration of CO in expired gas
$P(A-a)O_2$	Alveolar-arterial oxygen pressure difference; A-aDO$_2$ and $\Delta(A-a)PO_2$ has been used
SaO_2	Arterial oxygen saturation of hemoglobin
$\dot{Q}_s$	Shunt flow (total venous admixture) defined by the following equation:

$$\dot{Q}_s = \frac{CcO_2 - CaO_2}{CcO_2 - C\bar{v}O_2} \cdot Q$$

	Often expressed as a fraction of total flow.
$P_{ET}O_2$	PO$_2$ of end tidal expired gas
$(TCPO_2)$	Transcutaneous PO$_2$.

CONTRIBUTORS

Lee K. Brown, M.D.
Department of Medicine
Mount Sinai Medical Center
New York, New York

Roberta Goldring, M.D.
Department of Medicine
New York University Medical Center
New York, New York

David J. Kanarek, M.D.
Department of Medicine
Harvard Medical School
Boston, Massachusetts

Meyer Kattan, M.D.
Pediatric Pulmonary Center
Mount Sinai Medical Center
New York, New York

Albert Miller, M.D.
Director, Pulmonary Laboratory
Department of Medicine
Mount Sinai Medical Center
New York, New York

David M. Rapoport, M.D.
Department of Medicine
New York University Medical Center
New York, New York

E. Neil Schachter, M.D.
Director, Respiratory Therapy
Department of Medicine
Mount Sinai Medical Center
New York, New York

I. Barry Sorkin, M.D.
Department of Medicine
New York University School of Medicine
New York, New York

PULMONARY FUNCTION TESTS
A Guide for the Student and House Officer

Part I

Introduction

1

The Uses of Pulmonary Function Tests

Albert Miller

THE ROLE OF PULMONARY FUNCTION TESTS IN THE EVALUATION OF RESPIRATORY DISEASES

This book defines the *basic pulmonary function tests* as inspiratory and expiratory spirometry or flow-volume curves, full lung volumes, diffusing capacity, and arterial blood gases when indicated. In first evaluating patients with an actual (or suspected) respiratory problem, these tests constitute one of the three primary

PULMONARY FUNCTION TESTS: A   ISBN 0-8089-1764-4   Copyright © 1987 by Grune & Stratton
GUIDE FOR THE STUDENT AND HOUSE OFFICER   All rights of reproduction in any form reserved.

means to obtain data. The other two are the clinical examination (the medical history and the physical examination) and conventional chest roentgenography.

The data obtained from these three sources in the *individual patient* may then be supplemented or defined more precisely by specialized procedures such as fiberoptic bronchoscopy, bronchoalveolar lavage, thoracentesis, thoracoscopy, various biopsies, nuclear scans, computerized axial tomography, angiography, cardiac catheterization, and additional pulmonary function tests. These procedures are major advances in pulmonary diagnosis, but are utilized after a basic understanding of the patient's problems is achieved using the primary triad.

The relative contributions of the three elements of the respiratory triad vary with the clinical problem. Pulmonary function tests (with the possible exception of arterial gases) have little to add to the evaluation of an acute segmental or lobar pneumonia in an otherwise healthy patient, even though abnormal tests results may be obtained. The same may be said for a pleural effusion or "coin" lesion in the lung.

On the other hand, in early interstitial involvement of the lungs, pulmonary function tests may provide the only evidence of disease and thus the only indication for further evaluation. In asthma and in the clinical-pathologic mix that is variously referred to as chronic airways obstruction (CAO), chronic obstructive pulmonary disease (COPD), obstructive airways disease (OAD), etc., pulmonary function tests are more informative certainly than the chest film, and in most cases more than the clinical findings. In many instances, both the physician and the patient underestimate the severity of impairment.[1,2] This ignorance may contribute to the mortality and morbidity of obstructive airways disease.

THE CLINICAL APPLICATION OF PULMONARY FUNCTION TESTS

Identification of Primary Disease of the Respiratory System

The individual identified by abnormal pulmonary function tests frequently has no abnormal findings on clinical or radiographic examination. Examples include decreased vital capacity or diffusing capacity in a drug addict who injects talc crystals into his veins along with his intended drugs, or in a worker exposed to asbestos, or airways obstruction in a cigarette smoker or cotton mill worker.

Identification of Respiratory Involvement in a Systemic Disease or a Disease that Primarily Affects Another Organ System

This involvement can include restrictive impairment or diminished gas transfer in a patient with skin changes of scleroderma, or serologic changes suggestive of lupus erythematosus; or decreased vital capacity, maximal voluntary ventilation, or maximal respiratory force in a patient with neuromuscular disease.

THE USE OF PULMONARY FUNCTION TESTS
IN DIAGNOSIS

Patterns of Abnormality

It is frequently said that "pulmonary function tests do not establish a diagnosis." This is generally true, but in the same sense that radiography does not establish a diagnosis. The chest x-ray reveals patterns indicative of certain disease states, such as "a moderate-sized pleural effusion on the right side" or "a lobar consolidation." Some patterns are highly characteristic of common diseases and are therefore likely to be diagnostic, others are compatible with a long list of etiologically unrelated diseases with vastly different prognoses.

The radiographic presentation of diffuse interstitial infiltrates is no more "diagnostic" than the functional pattern of restrictive pulmonary impairment with diminished diffusion that frequently accompanies this presentation. Indeed, the histologic appearance on routine microscopic examination may be no more specific than the chest x-ray or pulmonary function tests. When a pathologist reports "usual interstitial pneumonitis" or "chronic inflammation and fibrosis," the patient may have a primary pulmonary disorder of unknown etiology or a multisystemic disease; the distinction is made by clinical and serologic findings. On the other hand, she may have a pneumoconiosis caused by the inhalation of particles not seen by the light microscope and detectable only by electron microscopic or mineralogic analysis.[3,4]

As in the case of radiographic patterns, pulmonary function patterns are consistent with certain diseases of varying etiology and natural history. What they have in common are their pathophysiologic pathways. The diagnostic significance of these patterns is discussed in Chapter 10.

Specific Patterns

The pattern of airways obstruction (decreased forced expiratory volume-1 second, decreased flows, increased airway resistance) is completely nonspecific and may be seen in emphysema and chronic bronchitis, recent or longstanding asthma, chemical or infectious insult to the airways, or pulmonary fibrosis with peribronchial involvement. However, this pattern together with a marked increase in residual volume, decrease in elastic recoil pressure, and decrease in diffusing capacity is more "diagnostic" of emphysema than any other set of clinical findings. On the other hand, this pattern together with normal elastic recoil and diffusing capacity and reversibility on bronchodilator administration is characteristic of asthma.

A positive response to provocation with a cholinergic agent or histamine establishes the presence of bronchial hyperreactivity, which in the absence of a predisposing factor such as respiratory infection, is considered a sufficent diagnosis to explain such nonspecific symptoms as chronic cough or episodic dyspnea.[5]

Primary alveolar hypoventilation may be cited as a diagnosis made by pulmonary function tests (even without evaluation of central nervous system responsiveness to respiratory stimuli). The diagnosis is established when retention of CO_2 is demonstrated despite normal mechanical and gas exchange properties of the lung, normal muscle force, and normal response to voluntary hyperventilation.

In a patient with alveolar-filling infiltrates, an increased diffusing capacity that soon falls from its elevated value may be a clue to pulmonary hemorrhage.

Use of Patterns to Exclude a Diagnosis

The absence of the expected physiologic findings does *not* exclude a diagnosis of ILD when it is suggested on radiographic or clinical grounds. The absence of airways obstruction at the time of testing does not eliminate asthma, but a negative response to provocation effectively rules out this diagnosis.

For practical purposes, chronic airways obstruction including emphysema is eliminated when airways obstruction is not demonstrated. We have reassured many patients who were referred to our laboratory with this diagnosis made on a routine radiographic examination. This is illustrated by Case Presentation 1-1, a 55-year-old nonsmoker with no symptoms whose chest roentgenogram (Figure 1-1), taken during a local Lung Association survey in 1971, was read as showing emphysema. Her (normal) pulmonary function studies at that time are detailed in Table 1-1. Twelve years later, she remained without evidence of CAO.

The problem is often elementary. Does a disorder of the respiratory system exist? If it does, can it explain the symptoms (usually dyspnea) in a patient with no or equivocal clinical and radiographic findings? Certainly, normal tests rule out CAO and a negative response to provocation rules out asthma. Normal lung volumes and gas exchange make interstitial fibrosis very unlikely if, as stated, the clinical and radiographic examinations are also negative. (Negative clinical and radiographic findings and normal lung volumes with *decreased D_LCO* suggest disease of the pulmonary vasculature.)

Patterns as an Indication for Invasive Procedures

Characteristic changes in pulmonary function tests are validly utilized to confirm the need for invasive procedures when clinical indications are insufficient. An example of this use of pulmonary function tests is to identify which patients at risk for the acquired immune deficiency syndrome (AIDS) to biopsy for opportunistic pulmonary infection. Early in the course of infection, symptoms may be slight and nonspecific, fever absent and the chest radiograph negative.

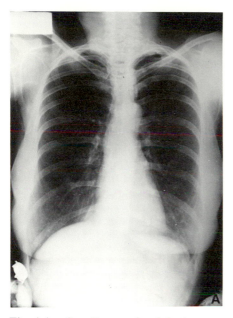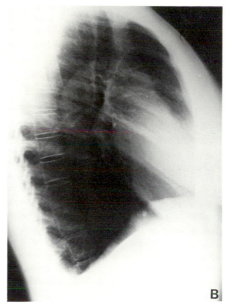

Fig. 1-1. Case Presentation 1-1. Apparent emphysema (radiographically). (A) PA projection shows hyperlucency, a vertical heart, and suggestive flattening of the diaphragm. (B) Lateral projection shows an increase in anteroposterior diameter and retrosternal air space. The subject, a 55-year-olds asymptomatic nonsmoker who had these films made during a local Lung Association screening program, was told she had emphysema. This was ruled out by the normal pulmonary function tests. In the ensuing 12 years, no clinical or physiologic evidence of CAO has been noted.

Table 1-1

Case Presentation 1-1, Radiographic "Emphysema" in a 55-Year-Old White Female Nonsmoker, 155 cm, 52.5 kg

Lung Volumes		Spirometry	
VC (cc)	3260(116%)*	FVC (cc)	3150(112%)
		FEV_1	2550(121%)
ERV	1150	FEV_1/FVC	0.81
FRC (He, MB)	2880	FEV_3/FVC	1.00
		$FEF_{200-1200}$(L/sec)	6.2
RV	1730(133%)	$FEF_{25-75\%}$	2.13(80%)
TLC	4990(121%)		
MVV (L/min)	83(122%)		
D_LCO_{SB} (cc/min/Torr)	21.0(100%)		

*In all Tables, values in parentheses are percent of predicted. Predicted values used in this book are Morris[11] or Miller's[12] reanalysis of Morris' data for spirometry, Miller[13] for D_LCO_{SB}, Baldwin. Cournand and Richards[14] for MVV and Goldman and Becklake[17] for VC/TLC ratio used to calculate TLC and RV from the VC predicted using Morris' data. Predicted values for lung volumes and FEV_1 of black subjects are reduced by 0.87.

In Case Presentation 1-2, the advent of abnormal test results, especially for D_LCO_{SB}, impelled the physician who had been treating a 40-year-old homosexual man for chronic cough to evaluate him more intensively. When the patient was first seen for this complaint in April 1982, clinical examination, chest radiograph and pulmonary function studies including methacholine provocation (Table 1-2) were virtually normal. Repeat testing in October demonstrated an 18 percent decrease in VC and a 76 percent decrease in D_LCO_{SB} from earlier values; the chest radiograph was equivocal. The patient was admitted to the hospital where transbronchial biopsy revealed *Pneumocystis carinii* and established the diagnosis of AIDS. Within one week, the radiograph showed bilateral confluent infiltrates (Figure 1-2). The patient responded to sulfamethoxazole-trimethoprim. Pulmonary function tests in March 1983 were improved but not normal. The patient died in August of that year with evidence of recurrent pneumocystis as well as *Mycobacterium intracellulare*.

Early Detection of Disease

It is well known that pulmonary function tests (especially D_LCO) may be abnormal before the clinical examination or chest x-ray is altered in the various interstitial lung diseases. For this reason, it is recommended that "patients with normal chest roentgenograms and normal mechanics of breathing but with impaired gas exchange should have lung biopsy for early diagnosis and therapy."[6] This

Table 1-2

Case Presentation 1-2, Advent of *Pneumocystis carinii* Pneumonia in a
40-Year-Old Black Male Nonsmoker with Chronic Cough, 173 cm, 73 kg

Lung Volumes	4/82		10/82
VC (cc)	3400(80%)*		2800(67%)
ERV	1320		900
FRC (plet)	3010		2510
RV	1690(89%)		1610(83%)
TLC	5170(84%)		4410(72%)
Spirometry		Methacholine (25 mg/cc)	
FVC (cc)	3400(80%)	3160, $\Delta = -7\%$	2610(62%)
FEV_1	3000(93%)	2810, $\Delta = -6\%$	2370(74%)
FEV_1/FVC	0.88		0.91
FEV_3/FVC	1.00		0.99
PFR (L/sec)	11.5		9.92
$FEF_{25-75\%}$	4.21(106%)		3.92(100%)
MVV (L/min)	153(125%)		142(124%)
D_LCO_{SB} (cc/min/Torr)	31.5(98%)		7.7(24%)
D_LCO/TLC_{SB}	6.23(125%)		2.01(41%)

*The 95 percent lower confidence limit is 82 percent of predicted.

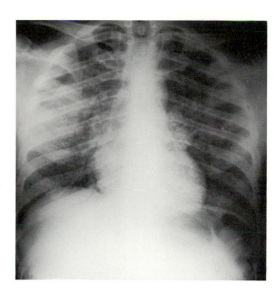

Fig. 1-2. Case Presentation 1-2. Acute interstitial pneumonitis due to *Pneumocystis carinii* in a 40-year-old black male with acquired immune deficiency syndrome. The chest film above shows a confluent finely nodular infiltrate. There has been a marked progression from subtle radiographic findings one week earlier, October 10, 1982, at which time a marked change was noted from previously normal pulmonary function in April, 1982. The decrease in lung volumes and marked decrease in D_LCO_{SB} were now characteristic of interstitial pneumonia.

important application of the D_LCO is discussed in greater detail in Chapter 7 and in the section on *Isolated Impairment in Diffusion* in Chapter 10.

Tests of small airways function are sensitive indicators of an effect on the lungs in populations at risk from environmental exposures. They are important in understanding the early natural history of CAO but are of little use in clinical decision making.

Pulmonary function tests often identify silent, clinically important CAO. Many patients who undergo routine spirometry (on physical examination, hospital admission, or preoperative evaluation, or during community or occupational screening) show severe obstructive impairment even though they are unaware of symptoms, or ascribe them to aging or cigarette smoking. Their physicians were similarly unaware of the presence of advanced disease.

Quantitation of Disease

Since pulmonary function tests are quantitative measurements, they are the most *objective* means to quantitate the extent of disease. It is more difficult to quantitate such clinical findings as dyspnea or quality of breath sounds or to standardize the reading of chest radiographs.

In general, pulmonary function tests correlate with the extent of disease demonstrated by clinical methods, including radiography. However, poor correlation with the conventional x-ray is well known in CAO and pulmonary vascular disease in which advanced disease may be unaccompanied by radiographic abnormalities, while patients with pneumoconiosis may present with dramatic x-rays and little impairment in lung function. Sarcoidosis may be cited as an example to prove both

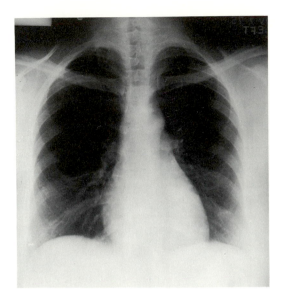

Fig. 1-3. Sarcoidosis in a dyspneic 40-year-old black female with a normal chest radiograph (stage "0") and positive Kveim test. The diffusing capacity is markedly decreased.

contentions. Looking at large numbers of patients, there is a correlation between degree and prevalence of impairment and the clinical-radiographic stage.[7] On the other hand, when studying individual patients, one finds frequent discrepancies. Extensive infiltrates may be seen on the x-ray with normal function while function may be markedly deranged with a normal x-ray (Stage 0, Figure 1-3, Table 1-3).

Much work has focused on the distinction between extent of *disease,* meaning disordered structure and function, and *activity* of the biologic processes underlying disease. We may again use sarcoidosis as an example of this distinction, since damage to the lungs is best assessed physiologically, while activity may be better correlated with cellular changes on broncho-alveolar lavage, with affinity for gallium-67 citrate on radioisotopic scanning, or with levels of certain enzymes (e.g., angiotensin converting enzyme or ACE) in serum or tissue. Many of these assessments are more costly, time consuming, hazardous, and/or invasive than conventional pulmonary function tests.

The following two uses of pulmonary function testing are applications of their quantitative nature.

Table 1-3
Sarcoidosis in a 40-Year-Old Black
Female Nonsmoker, 160 cm, 60 kg

FVC (cc)	2750 (93%)
FEV_1	2490 (108%)
FEV_1/FVC	0.91
$FEF_{25-75\%}$ (L/sec)	3.20 (100%)
MVV (L/min)	74 (88%)
D_LCO_{SB} (cc/min/Torr)	9.76 (42%)

FOLLOWING THE COURSE OF DISEASE

The various noninfectious interstitial lung diseases run variable courses. They may progress to a fatal outcome in a few months or remain stable for years. Pulmonary function tests are critical for elucidating these courses.

Most of the course of CAO is not clinically apparent; the diagnosis comes under consideration late in its long natural history. It is difficult to predict in the individual patient when respiratory failure is likely to occur. Serial pulmonary function tests will provide this information. From long-term longitudinal studies of patients with chronic bronchitis, it is apparent that a greater than expected decrease in pulmonary function (including as simple a test as FEV_1) offers the best guide to prognosis.[8] Even tests performed only once are informative. A low FEV_1 at age 40 years predicts that disabling disease will develop[9,10] while a value $\leq$ 800 cc portends CO_2 retention.

Similarly, in patients with chest bellows impairment of various types, surveillance of pulmonary function predicts the advent of respiratory insufficiency, which is usually the mode of death. This is true of a neuromuscular disease like amyotrophic lateral sclerosis (ALS), where precipitous decline in pulmonary function from normal levels may occur in the course of an illness lasting only several years. It is also true of a skeletal deformity like kyphoscoliosis, where a low level of pulmonary function may persist for many years with little change before deterioration is observed.

Indications for and Response to Therapy

For those diseases that significantly alter lung function, the decision whether to treat is guided by, and the results of treatment are monitored by, the measured changes in function. The clinician wants to know whether to begin treatment, whether to increase the dosage of an already prescribed medication, whether to prescribe additional or alternative drugs, or whether to advise further surgery following the initial procedure (eg, whether to operate on the opposite side for bullae or chronic fibrous pleurisy). Because of his close subjective relationship and his power of suggestion over patients with difficult diseases, the clinician requires objective quantitative guides in making these decisions. He will be misled if he relies solely on changes in symptoms or on such a subjective "quantitative" estimate as a clinical evaluation of the patient's exercise tolerance. In interstitial pneumonitis and in sarcoidosis, there is frequently a dissociation between improvement in clinical, radiographic, and physiologic indices. In CAO, the radiograph does not reflect response to treatment. In asthma, symptoms and signs may be misleading; monitoring a simple test like peak flow rate allows more precise adjustment of therapy. In all of these conditions, the most objective, quantitative, and pathophysiologically relevant indices of response are the pulmonary function tests.

References

1. McFadden ER Jr, Kiker R, DeGroot WJ: Acute bronchial asthma. N Engl J Med 288:221–225, 1973
2. Rubinfeld AR, Pain MC. How "mild" is mild asthma? Thorax 32:177–181, 1977
3. Miller A, Teirstein AS, Bader ME, et al. Talc pneumoconiosis: Significance of sublight microscopic mineral particles. Am J Med 50:395–402, 1971
4. Miller A, Langer AM, Teirstein AS, et al. Nonspecific interstitial pulmonary fibrosis: Association with asbestos fibers detected by electron microscopy. N Engl J Med 292:91–93, 1975
5. Corrao WM, Braman SS, Irwin RS. Chronic cough as the only presenting manifestation of bronchial asthma. N Engl J Med 300:633–637, 1979
6. Epler GR, McLoud TC, Gaensler EA, et al. Normal chest roentgenograms in chronic diffuse infiltrative lung disease. N Engl J Med 298:934–939, 1978
7. Miller A, Teirstein AS, Chuang MT. The sequence of physiologic changes in pulmonary sarcoidosis: Correlation with radiographic stages and response to therapy. Mt Sinai J Med 44:852–865, 1977
8. Bates DV. The fate of the chronic bronchitic: A report of the ten-year follow-up in the Canadian Department of Veteran's Affairs Coordinated study of chronic bronchitis. Am Rev Respir Dis 108:1043–1065, 1973
9. Fletcher C, Peto R, Tinker C, et al. The natural history of chronic bronchitis and emphysema: An eight year study of early chronic obstructive lung disease in working men in London. New York, Oxford University Press, 1976
10. Kronenberg RS, Niewoehner DE. Screening for early obstruction of the airways: A 1978 reappraisal (Editorial). Chest 74:610, 1978
11. Morris JF, Koski A, Johnson LC. Spirometric standards for healthy nonsmoking adults. Am Rev Respir Dis 103:57–67, 1971
12. Miller A, Thornton JC, Smith H Jr, et al. Spirometric "abnormality" in a normal male reference population: Further analysis of the 1971 Oregon Survey. Am J Indust Med 1:55–68, 1980
13. Miller A, Thornton JC, Warshaw R, et al. Single breath diffusing capacity in a representative sample of the population of Michigan, a large industrial state: Predicted values, lower limits of normal, and frequencies of abnormality by smoking history. Am Rev Respir Dis 127:270–277, 1983
14. Baldwin EF, Cournand A, Richards DW. Pulmonary insufficiency. I. Physiological classification, clinical methods of analysis, standard values in normal subjects. Medicine 27:243–278, 1948
15. Goldman HI, Becklake MR. Respiratory function tests. Normal values at median altitudes and the prediction of normal results. Am Rev Respir Dis 79:457–467, 1959

Part 11

Tests

2

Spirometry and Maximum Expiratory Flow-Volume Curves

Albert Miller

PULMONARY FUNCTION TESTS: A   ISBN 0-8089-1764-4   Copyright © 1987 by Grune & Stratton
GUIDE FOR THE STUDENT AND HOUSE OFFICER   All rights of reproduction in any form reserved.

INSTRUMENTATION

Spirometry is the measurement of volume change during various clearly defined breathing maneuvers. Using a volume displacement device (water-seal, rolling-seal, or wedge spirometer), expired (or inspired) volume is displayed against time in the classic *spirogram*. Recent instrumentation allows volume to be displayed against the simultaneous flow rate, thus producing a flow-volume (F-V) curve. Flow may be derived from the potentiometer signal of the spirometer or from a pneumotachygraph, whose flow signal is integrated to obtain volume.

MEASUREMENTS MADE FROM THE SPIROGRAM AND MEVF CURVE

Vital Capacity (VC) and Forced Vital Capacity (FVC)

Both the spirogram and the F-V curve are used to record the *same* basic expiratory maneuver, a maximum expiration made as rapidly as possible after a maximum inspiration. This is called the forced expiratory effort or *forced vital capacity (FVC) maneuver*. The spirogram is compared with the MEVF curve in Figure 2-1. The volume recorded during the forced expiratory maneuver is the forced *vital capacity,* meaning that the subject has been exhorted to expire as *rapidly,* in addition to as *completely,* as possible. When air trapping is present, the FVC is variably smaller than both the volume expired slowly after a maximum inspiration (the *slow* expiratory VC) and the volume inspired after a maximum, slow expiration (the *inspiratory* VC).

Expiratory Reserve Volume (ERV)

The ERV is the difference in volume between resting expiration (the end of a reproducible tidal volume) and forced expiration (the end of the VC maneuver). The resting expiratory level is the volume at which the inward recoil of the lungs is

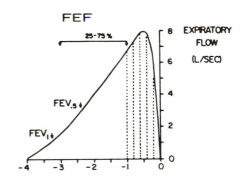

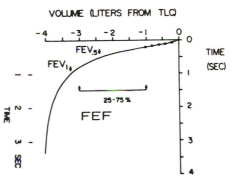

Fig. 2-1. Comparison of a spirogram with a MEFV curve. The vertical dashed lines indicate the
instantaneous flows at the expired
volumes shown in both curves. [Re-
produced from Hodgkin JE. Chronic
obstructive pulmonary disease. Chicago, American College of Chest
Physicians, 1979, p 25, with the
permission of the American College
of Chest Physicians.]

balanced by the outward recoil of the chest wall and both inspiratory and expiratory
muscles are at rest. The ERV in relation to the other lung volumes is illustrated in
Figure 2-2. The ERV is important in calculating *residual volume* (RV). Since
multiple breath dilution and plethysmography are most reproducible measured at the
resting level, the lung volume obtained from these procedures is the *functional
residual capacity* (FRC). It is necessary to subtract the ERV from the FRC to obtain
the RV.

The ERV is a useful measurement in itself. Normally, it is about one fifth to
two fifths of the VC (see Figure 2-2). It is reduced when excursion of the diaphragm
is limited and is a useful measurement in neuromuscular disease and in obesity,
where values below 400 cc were found to correlate with increased venous admixture
and arterial hypoxemia.[1]

Timed Forced Expiratory Volumes (FEV's)

One-Second (FEV₁)

The FEV₁ is the maximum volume that can be expired from a full inspiration in
one second. The FEV₁ may be considered a measurement both of volume and of

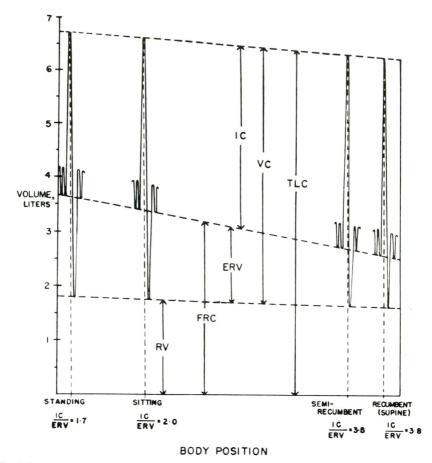

Fig. 2-2. Subdivisions of lung volume at various body positions as seen in the spirographic tracing at slow speed. [Reproduced from Boren HG, Kory RC, Snyder JC. The Veterans Administration-Army Cooperative Study of Pulmonary Function. II. The lung volume and its subdivisions in normal men. Am J Med 41:109, 1966, with permission.]

mean flow over the first second. It is frequently reported as a ratio to the FVC (the FEV_1/FVC *ratio*) or *one-second timed VC,* indicating the portion of the FVC that is expired in one second. While the FEV_1/FVC ratio is generally 0.70–0.80, ie, 70–80% of the FVC is expired in the first second in most subjects, this generalization is not always true. The relationship to this ratio of other factors such as sex, age, height, body build, and VC are discussed later in this chapter (*Factors Influencing Spirometric Results in Normal Subjects*).

The starting point for timing the FEV_1 is obtained by *backward extrapolation.*[2] The *zero time point* is determined by extending the steepest portion of the tracing

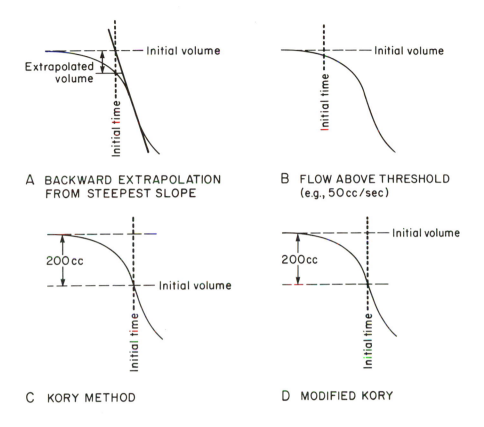

Fig. 2-3. Methods for calculating the FEV$_1$. Backward extrapolation (A) is the accepted standard; manual and computerized extrapolation provide similar results. Certain computer programs utilize a flow or volume threshold (B). Previous reference standards used the Kory (C) or modified Kory (D) methods.

(the maximum expiratory flow) back to the maximal inspiratory volume as illustrated in Figure 2-3. This compensates for a hesitant start. The extrapolated volume (the volume expired before time zero) must not exceed 10 percent of the FVC. Backward extrapolation is readily done by computer.

Three-Seconds (FEV$_3$)

The sensitivity of spirometry for detecting early air flow limitation is increased by analyzing the terminal portion of the forced expiration (after approximately two thirds of the FVC has been expired). The FEV$_3$ is a simple index of terminal events.

Standards for Acceptable Spirometric Tests

Instrumentation

Requirements for instrumentation have been standardized within the past decade by the American College of Chest Physicians[3,4] and the American Thoracic Society.[2] The spirometer should measure expired volumes up to 7 L and accumulate volume for at least 10 seconds. Resistance should be < 1.5 cm $H_2O/L/sec$ at a flow of 12 L/sec. Calibration is checked using a standard 3.0 L syringe.

All lung volumes and flow rates are reported *BTPS*, ie, at body temperature, ambient barometric pressure, and fully saturated with water vapor. The measurements made by a spirometer have been considered to be *ATPS*, ie, at ambient (room) temperature and conversion factors have been used to correct the measurements from ATPS to BTPS. These factors are shown in Table 2-1.

If the start of the FVC is the maximum inspiration and the start of the FEV_1 is defined by backward extrapolation, how is the *end* of the FVC maneuver defined? This is an important practical question since flow, and therefore volume, change is detectable for a long time in a subject with airflow obstruction. The FVC maneuver is considered at an end when the volume change is less than 25 cc or the flow rate is less than 0.05 L/sec within a half-second interval.[2] If this end point has not been reached, recording should continue for at least 10 seconds. Many spirograms recorded in the past were terminated before full expiration was reached.

A minimum of three acceptable FVC maneuvers must be obtained. An acceptable maneuver demonstrates a "crisp," unhesitating start; smooth, continuous expiration; absence of cough, glottis closure, second inspiration, leak (eg, at the mouthpiece), or blockage (eg, by the tongue); and complete effort. Early termination of effort can be easily missed and is discussed in more detail below. Both the FVC and FEV_1 of the best two of these three acceptable tracings must agree within 5 percent of the largest value or within 100 cc, whichever is greater.

The largest value for the FVC should be recorded as the FVC, and the largest value for the FEV_1 as the FEV_1, even if the two values do not come from the same effort. Provided the efforts agree within acceptable limits, there is little practical difference if one chooses one curve as the "best"[5] (see below) and reports all measurements from this, even if the FVC or FEV_1 is marginally larger on another effort.

Selection of the "Best Curve"

A workable definition of the best curve is that it have the largest sum of FVC and FEV_1 (and that the curve be acceptable in all the other ways outlined above). Reproducibility is demonstrated in Figure 2-4. When subjects are apprehensive, frightened, confused, or in pain, they are much less likely to comprehend the test and to perform maximally and reproducibly.

Table 2-1
Factors for Conversion of Volumes from
ATPS to STPD and BTPS (For BP 740–780)

Ambient Temperature (°C)	Water Vapor Pressure (Torr)	Appropriate Factor to Convert to	
		STPD	BTPS
10	9.2	0.952	1.153
11	9.8	0.949	1.148
12	10.5	0.945	1.143
13	11.2	0.940	1.138
14	12.0	0.936	1.133
15	12.8	0.932	1.128
16	13.6	0.928	1.123
17	14.5	0.924	1.118
18	15.5	0.920	1.113
19	16.5	0.916	1.108
20	17.5	0.911	1.102
21	18.7	0.906	1.096
22	19.8	0.902	1.091
23	21.1	0.897	1.085
24	22.4	0.893	1.080
25	23.8	0.888	1.075
26	25.2	0.883	1.069
27	26.7	0.878	1.063
28	28.3	0.874	1.057
29	30.0	0.869	1.051
30	31.8	0.864	1.045
31	33.7	0.859	1.039
32	35.7	0.853	1.032
33	37.7	0.848	1.026
34	39.9	0.843	1.020
35	42.2	0.838	1.014
36	44.6	0.832	1.007
37	47.1	0.826	1.000
38	49.7	0.821	0.994
39	52.4	0.816	0.987
40	55.3	0.810	0.980

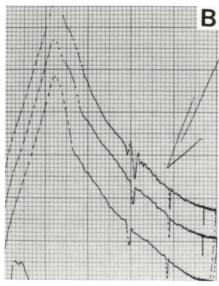

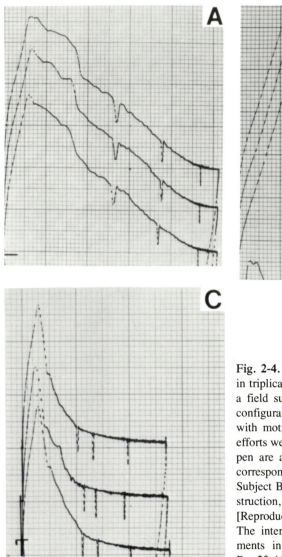

Fig. 2-4. (A–C) MEFV curves performed in triplicate by three consecutive subjects in a field survey, showing the consistency in configuration and results routinely obtained with motivated, well-coached subjects. *All* efforts were recorded. The deflections of the pen are at 0.5, 1.0, and 3.0 seconds and correspond to the $FEV_{0.5}$, FEV_1, and FEV_3. Subject B has changes of small airways obstruction, subject C, of airways obstruction. [Reproduced from Miller A, Thornton JC. The interpretation of spirometric measurements in epidemiologic surveys. Environ Res 23:448, 1980, with permission.]

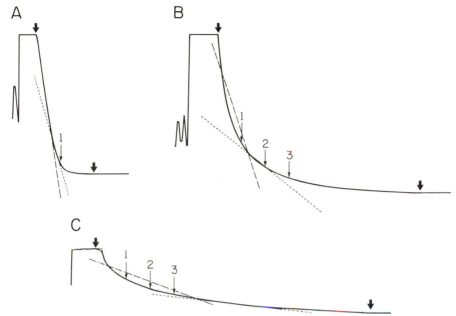

Fig. 2-5. Three spirograms showing calculation of $FEF_{25-75\%}$ and $FEF_{75-85\%}$ as well as FVC and FEV_{1-3}. (Redrawn from tracings using a water sealed spirometer and kymograph; volumes recorded ATPS). The FVC is delimited by the heavy arrows, the FEV_1, FEV_2, and FEV_3 are indicated by light arrows, the $FEF_{25-75\%}$ by long dashes, and the $FEF_{75-85\%}$ by short dashes. (A) was made by a healthy 27-year-old woman: FVC 3530 cc, FEV_1 3300 cc, FEV_3 3530 cc, $FEF_{25-75\%}$ 4.0 L/sec (virtually identical to the maximum flow), and $FEF_{75-85\%}$ 2.06 L/sec. (B) was made by a 30-year-old man whose asthma was in remission: FVC 4000 cc, FEV_1 2760 cc, FEV_3 3650 cc, $FEF_{25-75\%}$ 1.8 L/sec, and $FEF_{75-85\%}$, 0.5 L/sec. (C) was made by a 66-year-old woman with severe emphysema: FVC 1670 cc, FEV_1 950 cc (note backward extrapolation), FEV_3 1150 cc, $FEF_{25-75\%}$ 0.24 L/sec, and $FEF_{75-85\%}$ 0.06 L/sec.

Flow Rates

Flows Not Requiring a "Best Curve"

Obtained from the spirographic tracing: Maximum expiratory flow or forced expiratory flow $(FEF)_{200-1200}$. This is the flow rate at which the first liter of the FVC is expired. To eliminate the effect of a hesitant expiration, evidenced by a rounding of the spirographic tracing, the liter is measured after 200 cc have been expired. In a subject without airflow obstruction this part of the tracing is virtually a straight line (Figure 2-5). $FEF_{200-1200}$ is therefore very similar to peak flow rate (see immediately below).

Obtained from the MEFV curve (or from a pneumotachygraph or peak flow meter): Peak flow rate (PFR) or maximum forced expiratory flow (FEF max). This is the greatest expiratory flow measured.

It is often measured using a simple hand-carried "peak flow meter." This allows the patient to record it at home or on the job and quantitate the response to therapy, exercise, allergens, or occupational exposures.

Flows Requiring a "Best Curve" for Calculation

Obtained from the spirographic tracing: Maximum mid-expiratory flow (MMF) or forced expiratory flow (FEF)$_{25-75\%}$. To calculate this flow rate, the points on the spirogram at which 25 percent and 75 percent, respectively, of volume have been delivered are connected by a straight line, the slope of which (in L/sec) is the MMF (Figure 2-5). This is easily done graphically, or by a computer with memory. The volume is half (the "middle half") of the FVC and the time to deliver the specified volume is the *mid-expiratory time* (MET) *or forced expiratory time 25–75%* (FET$_{25-75\%}$).

The MMF is largely determined by the later, effort-independent part of the forced expiratory maneuver. Flow that is effort-independent is fixed in the sense that it will not increase with greater effort. (All spirometric measurements are "effort-dependent" in the sense that sufficient effort must be made to *reach* flow limitation and must be continued long enough to expire the full FVC.) For the past decade, flows at low lung volume, including the MMF, have been thought to be more specifically influenced by dimensional changes in the *small* airways and therefore, decreases in these flows have been thought to reflect small airways obstruction.

Although the concepts that underlie small airways obstruction are being re-thought, it is undeniable that many subjects who have normal values for FEV$_1$, FEV$_1$/FVC, and airways resistance have decreased values for MMF (and the other flow rates at low lung volume discussed in this section). These subjects are usually the very ones who are likely to have small airways obstruction, ie, cigarette smokers, workers exposed to irritant gases or fumes, or asthmatic patients in clinical remission. For patients with *clinical* evidence of airways disease, the decrement in MMF is usually greater than the decrement in FEV$_1$ or FEV$_1$/FVC.

The main difficulty in interpreting flow rates is that they are inherently more variable than FVC and FEV$_1$[6], with the result that the standard deviations (and the 95 percent confidence intervals) are a larger proportion of the predicted value. Indeed, when the predicted value is small (as in elderly or short or female subjects), the lower 95 percent confidence limit may be negative, which of course makes no physiologic sense. (See Chapter 9 for a fuller discussion of the 95 percent confidence interval.)

Mid-expiratory time (MET) or forced expiratory time (FET)$_{25-75\%}$. This measurement is not a flow; it is one axis of the MMF and is defined above. It is relatively independent of changes in lung volume and age and may therefore be easier to interpret. Leuallen and Fowler[7] reported normal values of 0.59 seconds in young men, 0.64 seconds in older men, and "about 0.5 seconds" in women. When it is not reported separately, the MET can be calculated from the FVC and MMF:

Equation 2-1

$$\text{MET (sec)} = \frac{\text{FVC (L)}}{2 \text{ MMF (L/sec)}}$$

Forced expiratory flow (FEF)$_{75-85\%}$.   Since flow is "averaged" at a lower lung volume than the middle half, namely over that 10 percent of the FVC starting at the point where 75 percent has been expired (Figure 2-5), this measurement was thought to be more sensitive in the detection of small airways obstruction. In actual use, it is often more difficult to measure and more affected by artifacts, like early termination of effort.

Obtained from the MEFV Curve: Instantaneous Flows

When flow is plotted against volume, instantaneous flow can be noted at any specified lung volume. The flow rate is called forced expiratory flow (FEF) when the reference volume is FVC and maximum flow ($\dot{V}$ max) when the reference volume is TLC. The specified volume is indicated by a subscript. The most commonly reported instantaneous flows are at 50 percent and 75 percent of FVC and at 60 percent of TLC. By consensus, these percentages refer to the volume of air *expired* when FVC is the reference, or *remaining in the lungs* when TLC is the reference. Thus, $\text{FEF}_{75\%}$ is the flow when 75 percent of the FVC has been expired while $\dot{V} \text{ max}_{60\%}$ is the flow when 60 percent of the TLC is still in the lungs (Figure 2-6).

Fig. 2-6.   The effects of inertia in the volume sensor and/or recording system on the MEFV curve, B, in a normal subject. Curve A is free of such effects. Note the lower and later peak flow and the apparent increase in flow in the middle volume range. The most commonly utilized instantaneous flows, at 50 and 75 percent of FVC and at 50 percent of TLC, are indicated. Less than maximal effort during the first part of the FVC would produce similar changes.

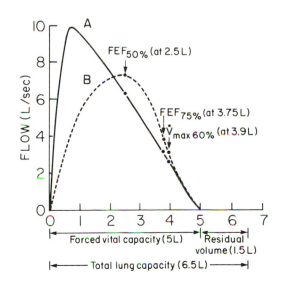

Instantaneous flows at low lung volumes (near or below FRC) are a simple means to detect small airways disease, but are fraught with difficulties. Their role in evaluating an individual patient is difficult to define. In the absence of clinical findings, reduced flows may be a clue to early disease. They help explain arterial hypoxemia in a patient without other abnormalities.

PERFORMANCE ARTIFACTS

Curves should be recorded whenever spirometry is performed; erroneous results brought about by improper or incomplete performance are often detectable.

Early termination of expiration is the most difficult artifact to recognize, since it occurs when most of the FVC has already been expired and its value may be reported as "normal." Early termination increases mean and instantaneous flow rates at middle and low lung volumes as well as the FEV_1/FVC. In subjects with normal values, the flow rates and flow-volume ratios calculated from such a tracing were seen to be unusually high. In some patients with clinical airflow obstruction, the degree of obstruction was underestimated, while in others, the values were those of restrictive rather than obstructive impairment.

In addition to detecting performance artifacts, MEFV curves provide a graphic demonstration of the type of impairment, eg, dynamic compression in emphysema, obstruction, small airways obstruction, restriction, etc. Certain normal variants are recognized, such as the "shoulder" seen in many healthy young men (Figure 2-7).

When superimposed on tidal inspiratory and expiratory loops, the maximum expiratory F-V curves also permit a dramatic—and semiquantitative—evaluation of ventilatory or flow "reserve." In a normal subject, the tidal loops occupy a very small area within the maximum. In a patient with emphysema (or upper airways obstruction), the tidal curves superimpose upon the maximum or even exceed it.

"Negative effort dependence" is a decrease in flows and FEV_1, and even in FVC, with maximal effort. It is usually due to dynamic compression of the airways in emphysema.

Figure 2-6 shows an artifact brought about by inertia in the instrumentation.

THE MATCH TEST

The ability to extinguish a lighted paper match held 6 inches from the open mouth correlates with $FEV_1 > 1.5$ L, $FEF_{200-1200} > 1.7$ L/sec, MMF > 0.6 L/sec, and MVV > 60 L/min. The reverse is less true, since a significant percentage of subjects with values greater than these failed to extinguish the match.[8]

PASSIVE SPIROMETRY

Ashutosh et al[9] described a method for obtaining spirometric measurements that requires no patient cooperation and can be performed on mechanically ventilated

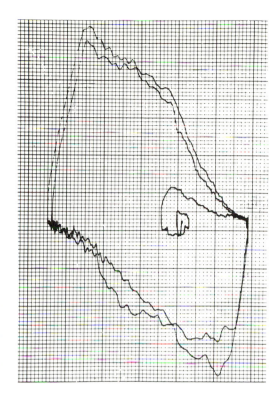

Fig. 2-7. A "shoulder" on the MEVF curve seen in many healthy young male subjects. Instead of progressively falling, flow is maintained during the first part of the FVC.

patients. The passive VC and passive expiratory volume-1 second are recorded from the expiratory circuit of a respirator set at a pressure limit of 30 cm H_2O. They correlated with the FEV_1 and FEV_1/FVC recorded at the same time.

FACTORS INFLUENCING SPIROMETRIC RESULTS IN NORMAL SUBJECTS

Age

It is well known that FVC, FEV_1, and flow rates in adults decline with age (see Chapter 9). Schoenberg et al[10] showed that FVC increases up to age 24 years and remains stable to age 35 years. Knudson et al[11] described three phases of spirometric function. Children (< 12 years of age) are in a *growth* phase; the dominant variable is height rather than age. *Maturation* begins with a growth spurt and continues until age 20 years in females and 25 years in males. Spirometric function is positively correlated with both age and height. Thereafter, during *decline*, measurements decrease with age.

It is less well recognized that FEV_1/FVC varies with age. Most cross-sectional surveys have shown a decline with age and then a slight increase in the elderly.[12-14] A five-year longitudinal study of 259 elderly subjects[15] disclosed a greater absolute and relative decline in FVC than in FEV_1 with a consequent increase in FEV_1/FVC. These changes were greater in men than women, and in those 70–90 years of age than in those 62–69 years of age.

Height

Conversion between metric and English units of height and weight is shown in Table 2-2. All spirometric measurements increase with body size, which is generally the only variable in predictive equations for children. In adults, the correlation with overall height is generally as good as with other indices of body size, such as powers of height or multiples of height and weight. The best correlation would seem to be with trunk length or sitting height, since differences in spirometric values between racial groups have been explained by different ratios between trunk and lower extremity length (See *Race*, below).

Although all spirometric measurements increase with height, FVC increases more than FEV_1 or flows. This may result from an increase in number and/or size of alveoli relative to airways so that "larger lungs are likely to take longer to empty than smaller ones."[16] It has been our observation that many subjects who are more than 75 inches tall have FVC values considerably above the predicted, while FEV_1 values are in the expected range. These tall, healthy nonsmokers may have FEV_1/FVC values lower than expected. If FEV_1/FVC is the only criterion considered, they would be diagnosed as having airways obstruction. Several workers have confirmed that FEV_1/FVC is negatively correlated with FVC.

For subjects whose height cannot be measured (eg, they are unable to stand or have severe skeletal deformities such as kyphoscoliosis), height is very similar to arm span.[17] Using this calculated height rather than actual height to predict pulmonary function values in kyphoscoliosis results in larger predicted values and demonstrates more clearly the physiologic impairments.

Table 2-2
Conversion of Units of Height and Weight

English	Metric
1 inch	2.54 cm
0.394 inch	1 cm
1 pound (lb)	0.454 kg
2.205 lb	1 kg

Body surface area $(M^2) = Kg^{0.425} \times cm^{0.725} \times 7.184 \times 10^{-3}$

Weight

Spirometric results are positively correlated with weight to the extent that increased weight means growth or muscle mass. Beyond this (ie, with obesity), spirometric values (and lung volumes, especially ERV) decrease with greater weight.

Body Position

The effects of change in body position on lung volumes are illustrated in Figure 2-2. They are caused by greater ability of the diaphragm to descend in the standing compared with the seated and especially the supine positions.

Muscular Development

There is evidence that certain athletes[18,19] and those persons such as divers and miners, whose work activities develop the pectoral muscles (including the accessory muscles of respiration) have a relatively greater FVC compared to FEV_1, with a correspondingly lower FEV_1/FVC.[20]

Respiratory pressures, a test of respiratory muscle strength, were found to be the main determinant (after height) of FVC, FEV_1, and PFR in both sexes, in a study of 924 healthy white subjects 13–35 years of age.[21] In this age span, age had no effect. The effect of muscle wasting and nutritional depletion on spirometric performance is well known.

Race

Blacks residing both in Africa and in the New World[22-37] have smaller height coefficients for lung volumes and generally for flows than do whites. Indians and Pakistanis, wherever resident,[38-47] Orientals,[33,48-52] Pacific Islanders,[53-57] and North American Indians are generally intermediate between whites and blacks.

This knowledge has not consistently been applied in the clinical interpretation of pulmonary function tests. Since most studies have shown the difference in FVC and FEV_1 for black adults to be in the range of 10–20 percent, a 13 percent scaling factor has been proposed to adjust the values predicted for whites.[58] Values for FEV_1/FVC in blacks are generally higher than in whites.[36]

Sex

Most pulmonary function values are lower in women, even when adjustments are made for differences in size. The FEV_1/FVC is higher. Knudson[11] found that FVC and FEV_1 started to decline at an earlier age in women (20 years) than in men (25 years).

References

1. Holley HS, Milic-Emili J, Becklake MR, et al. Regional distribution of pulmonary ventilation and perfusion in obesity. J Clin Invest 46:475–481, 1967
2. Ferris BG (Principal Investigator). Epidemiology standardization project. Am Rev Respir Dis 118, Part 2, 1978
3. American College of Chest Physicians, Committee Recommendations. The assessment of ventilatory capacity. Statement of the Committees on Environmental Health and Respiratory Physiology. Chest 67:95–97, 1975
4. American College of Chest Physicians. Scientific Section Recommendations. Statement on spirometry: A report of the section on respiratory pathophysiology. Chest 83:547–550, 1983
5. Sorensen JB, Morris AH, Crapo RO, et al. Selection of the best spirometric values for interpretation. Am Rev Resp Dis 122:802–805, 1980
6. Rozas CJ, Goldman, AL. Daily spirometric variability: Normal subjects and subjects with chronic bronchitis with and without air flow obstruction. Arch Intern Med 142:1287–1291, 1982
7. Leuallen EC, Fowler WS. Maximal midexpiratory flow. Amer Rev Tuberc 72:783–800, 1955
8. Dines DE, Fowler WS. Chronic obstructive airway disease: Comparison of match test and vitalor with standard pulmonary function tests. Minn Med 51:33–36, 1968
9. Ashutosh K, Auchincloss JH Jr, Gibert R. Passive spirometry used to evaluate pulmonary function in patients receiving mechanical assistance to ventilation. Chest 68:645–650, 1975
10. Schoenberg JB, Beck GJ, Bouhuys A. Growth and decay of pulmonary function in healthy blacks and whites. Resp Physiol 33:367–393, 1978
11. Knudson JF, Lebowitz MD, Halberg CJ, et al. Changes in the normal maximal expiratory flow-volume curve with growth and aging. Am Rev Resp Dis 127:725–734, 1983
12. Morris JF, Temple WP, Koski A. Normal values for the ratio of one-second forced expiratory volume to forced vital capacity. Am Rev Resp Dis 108:1000–1003, 1973
13. Schmidt CD, Dickman ML, Gardner RM, et al. Spirometric standards for healthy elderly men and women: 532 subjects, ages 55 through 94 years. Am Rev Resp Dis 108:933–939, 1973
14. Higgins MW, Keller JB. Seven measures of ventilatory lung function. Population values and a comparison of their ability to discriminate between persons with and without chronic respiratory symptoms and disease, Tecumseh, Michigan. Am Rev Resp Dis 108:258–272, 1973
15. Milne JS. Longitudinal respiratory studies in older poeple. Thorax 33:547–554, 1978
16. Burrows B, Cline MG, Knudson RJ, et al. A descriptive analysis of the growth and decline of the FVC and FEV_1. Chest 83:717–724, 1983
17. Hepper NGG, Black LF, Fowler WS. Relationships of lung volume to height and arm span in normal subjects and in patients with spinal deformity. Am Rev Resp Dis 91:356–362, 1965
18. Shapiro W, Johnston CE, Dameron RA Jr, et al. Maximum ventilatory performance and its limiting factors. J Appl Physiol 19:199–203, 1964
19. Shapiro W, Patterson JF Jr. Effects of smoking and athletic conditioning on ventilatory mechanics including observations on the reliability of the forced expirogram. Am Rev Resp Dis 85:191–199, 1962

20. Jain BL, Patrick JM. Ventilatory function in Nigerian miners. Br J Industr Med 38:275–280, 1981

21. Leech JA, Ghezzo H, Stevens D, et al. Respiratory pressures and function in young adults. Am Rev Resp Dis 128:17–23, 1983

22. Smillie WG, Augustine DL. Vital capacity of negro race. JAMA 87:2055–2058, 1926

23. Roberts FI, Crabtree JA. The vital capacity of the negro child. JAMA 25:1950–1952, 1927

24. Abramowitz S, Leiner GC, Lewis WA, et al. Vital capacity in the negro. Am Rev Resp Dis 92:287–292, 1965

25. Damon A. Negro-White differences in pulmonary function (vital capacity, timed vital capacity, and expiratory flow rate). Hum Biol 38:380–393, 1966

26. Johannsen ZM, Erasmus LD. Clinical Spirometry in normal Bantu. Am Rev Resp Dis 97:585–597, 1968

27. Hearn CED. Bagassosis. An epidemiological, environmental and clinical survey. Br J Industr Med 25:267–282, 1968

28. Densen PM, Jones EW, Bass HE, et al. A survey of respiratory disease among New York City postal and transit workers. II. Ventilatory function test results. Environ Res 2:277–296, 1969

29. Oduntan SA. Spirometric studies of normal preoperative patients in Nigeria. African J Med Sci 1:79–84, 1970

30. Femi-Pearse D, Elebeute EA. Ventilatory function in healthy adult Nigerians. Clin Sci 41:203–211, 1971

31. Miller GJ, Cotes JR, Hall AM, et al. Lung function and exercise performance of healthy Caribbean men and women of African ethnic origin. Q J Exp Physiol 57:325–341, 1972

32. Lapp NL, Amandus HE, Hall R, et al. Lung volumes and flow rates in black and white subjects. Thorax 29:185–188, 1974

33. Seltzer CC, Siegelaub AB, Friedman GD, et al. Differences in pulmonary function related to smoking habits and race. Am Rev Resp Dis 110:598–608, 1974

34. Binder RE, Mitchell CA, Schoenberg JB, et al. Lung function among black and white children. Am Rev Resp Dis 114:955–959, 1976

35. Mustafa KY. Spirometric lung function tests in normal men of African ethnic origin. Am Rev Resp Dis 116:209–213, 1977

36. Lanese RR, Keller MD, Foley MF, et al. Differences in pulmonary function tests among Whites, Blacks and American Indians in a textile company. J Occup Med 20:39–44, 1978

37. Stinson JM, McPherson GL, Hicks K, et al. Spirometric standards for healthy black adults. J Nat Med Assoc 73:729–733, 1981

38. Williams DE, Miller RD, Taylor WF. Pulmonary function studies in healthy Pakistani adults. Thorax 33:243–249, 1978

39. Mason ED. Standards for predicting the normal vital capacity of the lungs in south Indian women from height, weight and surface area. Indian J Med Res 20:117–134, 1932–1933

40. Rao MN, Sen Gupta A, Saha PN, et al. Physiological norms of Indians: Pulmonary capacities in health. Indian Council of Medical Research Special Report Series, No. 38, New Delhi, 1961

41. Raghaven P, Nagendra AS. A study of ventilatory functions in healthy Indian adults. J Postgrad Med (Bombay) 11:99–108, 1065

42. Cotes JE, Malhotra MS. Differences in lung function between Indians and Europeans. J Physiol (Lond) 177:17P–18P, 1965

43. Bhattacharya AK, Banerjee S. Vital capacity in children and young adults in India. Ind J Med Res 54:62–71, 1966

44. Jain SK, Ramiah TJ. Influence of age, height and body surface area on lung functions in healthy women 15–40 years old. Indian J Chest Dis 9:13–22, 1967

45. Jain SK, Ramiah TJ. Normal standards of pulmonary function tests for healthy Indian men 15–40 years old: Comparison of different regression equations (prediction formulae). Indian J Med Res 57:1453–1466, 1969

46. Malik MA, Moss E, Lee WR. Prediction values for the ventilatory capacity in male West Pakistani workers in the United Kingdom. Thorax 27:611–619, 1972

47. Corey PN, Ashley MJ, Chan-Yeung MB. Racial differences in lung function. Search for proportional relationships. J Occup Med 21:395–398, 1979

48. Foster JH. A study of vital capacity of Chinese. China Med J 38:285–294, 1924

49. Wu MC, Yang SP. Pulmonary function study in healthy Chinese. I. Lung volume and its subdivisions. J Formosan Med Assoc 61:110–129, 1962

50. Cotes JE, Ward MP. Ventilatory capacity in normal Bhutanese. Physiology 186:88P–89P, 1966

51. Da Costa JL. Pulmonary function studies in healthy Chinese adults in Singapore. Am Rev Resp Dis 104:128–131, 1971

52. Chin B, Horsfall PAL. Lung volumes in normal Cantonese subjects. Preliminary studies. Thorax 32:352–355, 1977

53. Glass WI. Ventilatory function differences between Polynesian and European rope workers. NZ Med J 61:433–444, 1962

54. Dugdale AE, Bolton JM, Ganendran A. Respiratory function among Malaysian aboriginals. Thorax 26:740–743, 1971

55. Woolcock AJ, Colman MH, Blackburn CRB. Factors affecting normal values for ventilatory lung function. Am Rev Resp Dis 106:692–709, 1972

56. Cotes JE, Anderson HR, Patrick JM. Lung function in response to exercise in New Guineans: Role of genetic and environmental factors. Philos Trans R Soc London 268:349–361, 1974

57. Brown P, Sadowsky D, Gajdusek DC. Ventilatory lung function measurements in Pacific Island Micronesians. Amer J Epidemiol 108:259–265, 1978

58. Rossiter CE, Weill H. Ethnic differences in lung function. Evidence for proportional differences. Int J Epidemiol 3:55–61, 1974. Spirometric changes in normal children with upper respiratory infections. Am Rev Resp Dis 117:47–53, 1978

3

Inspiratory Flows and Flow-Volume Loops in the Diagnosis of Upper Airways Obstruction

Albert Miller

Types of Upper Airways Obstruction (UAO) Recognized by Flow-Volume Loops
  Fixed UAO
    Physiologic Findings
    Causes
  Variable UAO
    Extrathoracic
    Intrathoracic
Coexisting Lower Airways Obstruction
  Masking Lower Airways Obstruction in the Presence of UAO
  Masking UAO in the Presence of Lower Airways Obstruction

    The inspiratory flow-volume loop should be recorded on every patient. Depending on the degree of clinical suspicion of such a lesion, it can provide the first *clue* or the most easily obtained *confirmation* of an obstructive process in the trachea, larynx, or pharnyx.

    Upper airway obstruction is increasingly being recognized. This is partly due to increased awareness on the part of clinicians but also represents an increase in the number of cases brought about by tracheal intubation with cuffed tubes. Astute clinicians are aware that "all that wheezes is not asthma." Increasingly, patients with labored, noisy breathing who had been diagnosed and treated as asthma are recognized to have obstruction in the upper airways or main bronchi.

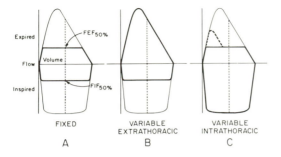

Fig. 3-1. Characteristic flow-volume loops in the three types of UAO commonly described. Normal loops are superimposed with a light line.

TYPES OF UPPER AIRWAYS OBSTRUCTION (UAO) RECOGNIZED BY FLOW-VOLUME LOOPS

The typical physiologic changes seen in each type are described below and the characteristic F-V loops illustrated in Figure 3-1. It should be borne in mind that the pathologic correlation with these physiologic patterns is not precise. Stenoses, tumors, and compression often result in overlapping findings. The classification was proposed by Miller and Hyatt in 1969 and 1973.[1,2] They also determined the degree of narrowing necessary to produce UAO by inserting progressively smaller orifices in the breathing circuit of normal volunteers. The PFR and MVV were the most sensitive measurements; FEV_1 did not decrease until the orifice was reduced to 6 mm in diameter. These changes are shown in Figure 3-2; F-V plots of one subject are shown in Figure 3-3.

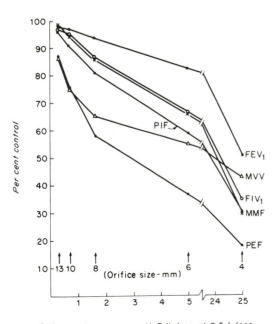

Fig. 3-2. Inspiratory and expiratory flows plotted against the resistance imposed by a progressively narrower breathing circuit. Flows are shown as percentages of control values. Subjects were seven normal males. Compare with Figure 3-9. [From Miller RD, Hyatt RE. Obstructing lesions of the larnyx and trachea: Clinical and physiologic characteristics. Mayo Clin Proc 44:147, 1969, with permission.]

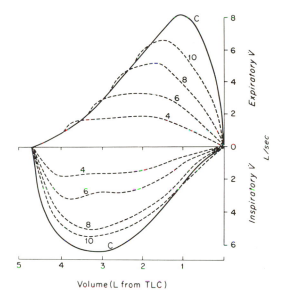

Fig. 3-3. Flow-volume loops when increasingly severe UAO was imposed on a normal subject by breathing through progressively smaller external orifices. The unobstructed loops are shown by the unbroken line. [From Miller RD, Hyatt RE. Obstructing lesions of the larnyx and trachea: Clinical and physiologic characteristics. Mayo Clin Proc 44:148, 1969, with permission.]

Fixed UAO

Physiologic Findings

The term "fixed" does not have the same meaning as it does when applied to lower airways obstruction, in which it implies irreversibility because of lack of response to a bronchodilator. With a fixed obstruction in the upper airways, the airway diameter at the site of the lesion does not change with inspiratory or expiratory effort. There is an increased resistance to flow that remains constant during both phases of the respiratory cycle, resulting in plateaus during inspiration and expiration. A plateau is obvious as a straight line (indicating constant flow), which is horizontal on F-V curves and diagonal on the spirogram. Since both inspiration and expiration are affected, the ratio of inspiratory to expiratory flow at mid-VC ($FIF_{50\%}/FEF_{50\%}$) may not change from its normal value (≥ 1.0); peak flow is especially diminished. On spirometry, the normal exponential expiratory curve is lost, the inspiratory and expiratory limbs of the spirogram resemble each other and FEV_1 is about the same as the one second forced inspiratory volume (FIV_1).

Causes

Postintubation stenosis. Lesions that cause fixed UAO are usually circumferential. The most common lesion is postintubation cicatricial stenosis of the trachea. Endotracheal intubation generally causes edema, hemorrhage, and then fibrosis and damage to the cartilage at the cuff site in the intrathoracic trachea; tracheostomy lesions are in the extrathoracic trachea.

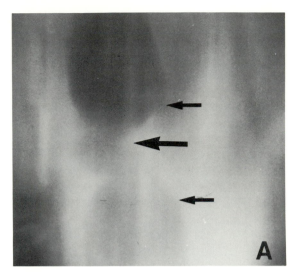
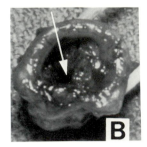

Fig. 3-4. (A) Frontal tomogram of the neck showing a localized stenosis encircling the upper trachea. The longer arrow indicates the greatest narrowing, the two smaller arrows, the extent of the stenosis (two rings). (B) Surgical resection of trachea showing circumferential cicatricial stenosis; the extremely compromised lumen is shown by the arrow. [Courtesy of Dr. Peter M. Som, Radiology Department, Mt Sinai Medical Center, New York.]

Figure 3-4 shows the tomogram of the air column in the neck (A) demonstrating a localized stenosis that was excised (B). In the more extensive obstruction shown in Figure 3-5, necrosis of the mucosa, submucosa, and cartilage involves several tracheal rings.

Case Presentation 3-1 is a 19-year-old female nonsmoker who underwent prolonged open heart surgery at age 8 years in 1966 for correction of a Tetralogy of Fallot. This was followed by a long period of intensive care with a tracheostomy in place. Symptoms of loud and labored breathing on exertion led to her evaluation in a pulmonary function laboratory in 1977; results are shown in Table 3-1. These show normal lung volumes, moderate reduction in FEV_1 and in all flows on expiration and inspiration, and a marked reduction in MVV. Further workup was refused by the patient, who chose to avoid those activities that produced her symptoms. Repeat studies two and six years later showed some improvement in FEV_1 and MVV. Flow-volume loops characteristic of fixed UAO are shown in Figure 3-6.

Goiters. The trachea is occasionally encircled from without by goiters, causing UAO.

Endotracheal neoplasms. Neoplasms such as oat cell carcinomas primary in the trachea[3] or invading from a main bronchus can cause encirclement from within.

Stenosis of both main bronchi. We have described two cases in which narrowing of both main bronchi produced the characteristic findings of fixed UAO.[4]

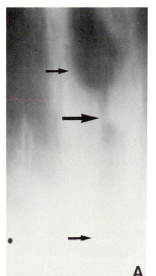 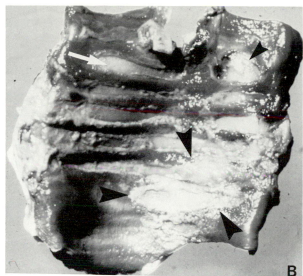

Fig. 3-5. (A) Frontal tomogram of the neck showing an extensive posttracheostomy stenosis involving six rings. The larger arrow indicates the greatest narrowing, the smaller arrows the extent of the stenosis. The film is less magnified than that in Figure 3A. (B) Necropsy specimen showing varying degrees of cuff injury. The white arrow indicates ulceration overlying a ring cartilage, the area most susceptible to pressure necrosis. The smaller black arrow indicates ulceration over two rings and their intercartilaginous membrane. The larger black arrows indicate an extensive ulcer with fragmented cartilage at its base. The tracheostomy opening is seen in the upper margin of the specimen. [From Som PM, Khilnani MT, Keller RJ, et al. Tracheal stenosis secondary to cuffed tubes. Mt. Sinai J Med 40:654, 1973, with permission.]

Case Presentation 3-2, included in this report, is a 32-year-old black woman with florid sarcoidosis of the skin and peripheral and mediastinal lymphadenopathy (positive biopsies) of three years' duration. Wheezing and dyspnea had progressed over a two-year period. The patient was in respiratory distress, with evident stridor. Bilateral hilar adenopathy and minor diffuse infiltrates were seen on the chest film. Frontal tomograms (Fig. 3-7A) of the chest showed symmetrical stenosis of both main bronchi with noncritical narrowing of the distal trachea. Rigid bronchoscopy demonstrated erythema and swelling of the tracheal and bronchial mucosae, with marked narrowing of the main bronchi.

Pulmonary function results (Table 3-2) showed a normal FVC, and marked reductions in FEV_1, FEV_3, inspiratory and expiratory flows, and MVV. The F-V loops (Fig. 3-7B) were characteristic of fixed UAO.

Obstruction of the external airway. Fixed obstruction is seen in the intensive care unit when the patient breathes through an occluded or inappropriately small endotracheal tube. It is produced at will in the laboratory in order to investigate the

Table 3-1*

Case Presentation 3-1, Posttracheostomy Tracheal Stenosis, 19-Year-Old White Female Nonsmoker, 165 cm, 69 kg

Lung Volumes	8/77	7/79	5/83
VC (cc)		3700(90%)	
ERV		1150	
FRC (plet)		2370	
RV		1220(78%)	
TLC		4920(86%)	
Spirometry and Flows			
FCV (cc)	3700(104%)	3690(90%)	3700(93%)
FEV_1	1870(56%)	2280(69%)	2280(71%)
FEV_1/FVC	0.51	0.62	0.62
PFR (L/sec)		2.7	2.6
$FEF_{25-75\%}$		2.1(55%)	2.0(54%)
$FEF_{50\%}$	1.86	2.4	2.3
$FIF_{50\%}$		2.0	1.9
MVV (L/min)	36(32%)	52(58%)	
D_LCO_{SB} (cc/min/Torr)		20.5(78%)	

*See footnote to Table 1-1, page 7, for description of predicted values used for tables showing pulmonary function test results.

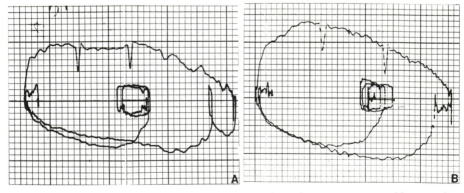

Fig. 3-6. Case Presentation 3-1 (A) Maximum F-V loops in a young woman 11 years after prolonged tracheostomy following correction of Tetralogy of Fallot. Symmetrical inspiratory and expiratory curves are characteristic of fixed UAO; tests performed when patient dyspneic, with obvious stridor. (B) Curves three years later; patient comfortable, stridor less apparent. In both graphs, one large division equals one liter of volume and 2 L/sec of flow.

Table 3-2

Case Presentation 3-2, Fixed UAO
Associated with Bilateral Stenosis of the
Main Bronchi Secondary to Sarcoidosis in
a 32-Year-Old Black Female Exsmoker,
169 cm, 86 kg

FVC (cc)	2820 (81%)
FEV_1	720 (26%)
FEV_1/FVC	0.25
FEV_3/FVC	0.59
$FEF_{25-75\%}$ (L/sec)	0.42 (12%)
$FEF_{50\%}$	0.62
$FIF_{50\%}$	0.80
MVV (L/min)	21 (19%)
D_LCO_{SB} (cc/min/Torr)	29.8 (116%)

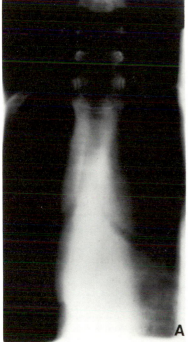

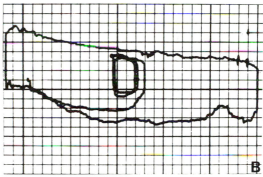

Fig. 3-7. (A) Case Presentation 3-2. Frontal tomogram of a 32-year-old woman showing symmetrical narrowing of both main bronchi most
marked proximally, as well as lesser narrowing of
the distal trachea. Paratracheal and hilar lymphadenopathy can be made out. Previous medias-
tinoscopy confirmed sarcoidosis. (B) Maximum
flow volume loops in the same patient characteristic of fixed UAO. One large division equals one
liter of volume and 2 L/sec of flow.

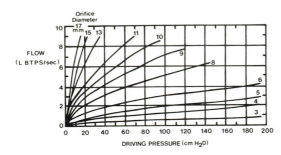

Fig. 3-8. Estimation of airway diameter from flow ($FEF_{50\%}$ or $FIF_{50\%}$); driving pressure is assumed to be between 50 and 150 cm H_2O. Curve was constructed by using graded external resistances in a normal subject. [From Gamsu G, Borson DB, Webb WR, et al. Structure and function in tracheal stenosis. Am Rev Resp Dis 121:530, 1980, with permission.]

mechanics of airflow, by breathing through progressive narrowings in the external airway (Fig. 3-3). Such studies permit estimation of the diameter of a stenotic lesion from the patient's F-V loops.[5] From Figure 3-8, it may be seen that if $FEF_{50\%}$ (or $FIF_{50\%}$) is 2.5 L/sec, the diameter is 5.5 mm (assuming a driving pressure of about 100 cm H_2O).

Variable UAO

The term "variable" means that the obstruction follows the dynamics of flow and pressure during the respiratory cycle. The lesion may itself be "variable" in the sense of *mobile* or even *floppy* as in vocal cord paralysis, tracheomalacia, or relapsing polychrondritis, or it may be quite unchanging, such as an intraluminal tumor.[6,7] Such projecting lesions are localized rather than circumferential and produce obstruction by creating a crescentic lumen, the remainder of which is the normal compliant wall of the airway.

Extrathoracic

Physiologic findings.   During inspiration, the pressure within the extrathoracic (defined as more than 2 cm above the manubrium[2]) airway is negative compared to the atmospheric pressure around it. When an obstructing lesion is present, the further decrease in diameter on inspiration results in a flow plateau. During expiration, positive pressure within the airway widens the lumen and the expiratory loop is unchanged from what it would be otherwise. The characteristic flow-volume loops are shown in Figure 3-1B. The ratio of $FIF_{50\%}$ to $FEF_{50\%}$ (or MMIF to MMEF) is decreased and FEV_1 is greater than FIV_1.

Causes: Bilateral vocal cord paralysis.   The lateral diameter in the larynx may be < 2 mm.

Unilateral vocal cord paralysis.   This is a more common lesion and may also result in UAO. Cormier[8] reported 15 cases. In the 10 patients who underwent reconstruction, $FIF_{50\%}$ increased while $FEF_{50\%}$ did not change. Case Presentation

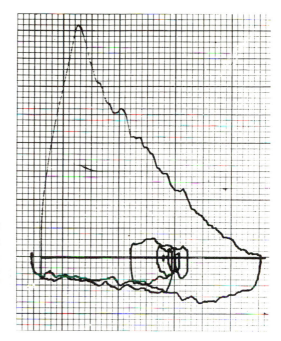

Fig. 3-9. Case Presentation 3-3. Maximum F-V loops characteristic of variable extrathoracic obstruction in a 47-year-old man with unilateral vocal cord paralysis due to extensive tumor involvement (Schwanoma) of cranial nerves. One large division equals one liter of volume and 2 L/sec of flow.

3-3 is a 47-year-old white man who noted a change in his voice for more than one year followed by difficulty swallowing. Laryngyoscopy revealed a unilateral left vocal cord paralysis, which proved secondary to a Schwanoma of the tenth cranial nerve at the base of the brain, extending to the twelfth nerve. The pulmonary function data showed normal FVC and expiratory flows, with marked reductions in inspiratory flow and MVV. The F-V loops are seen in Figure 3-9.

Adhesions of the vocal cords.   These result from abrasion of the cords during endotracheal intubation, especially when this is performed as an emergency procedure.

Vocal cord constriction.   Intermittent obstruction has been observed in patients with recurrent inspiratory stridor and no anatomic abnormalities. Flow-volume curves when symptoms were not present were normal.[9,10] Constriction of the vocal cords was documented during attacks by indirect laryngoscopy or by fiberoptic endoscopy and videorecording.

Obstructive sleep apnea.   Flow-volume curves may be useful in evaluating sleep disordered breathing. Of 35 patients with obstructive sleep apnea, 14 (40 percent) showed variable extrathoracic obstruction.[11] Sanders[12] described "sawtoothing" on the inspiratory and/or expiratory F-V loop (Figure 3-10).

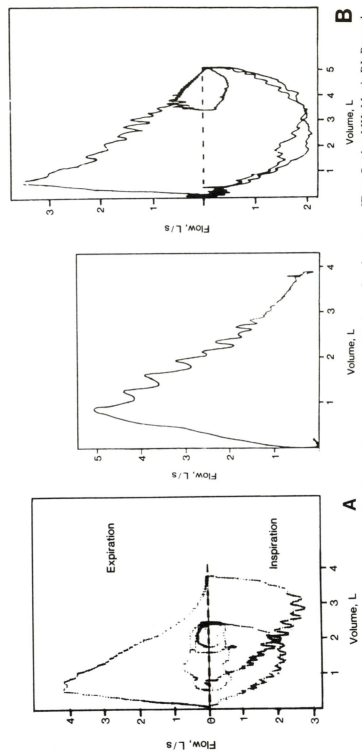

Fig. 3-10. "Sawtoothing," on inspiratory (A) and expiratory (B) loops of patients with obstructive sleep apnea. [From Sanders MH, Martin RJ, Pennock BE, et al. The detection of sleep apnea in the awake patient. The "saw tooth" sign. JAMA 245:2415 and 2417, 1981, with permission.]

Burns. In a recent study[13] of burn patients *without* clinically evident UAO (e.g., stridor), almost half showed variable extrathoracic obstruction. This correlated with the severity of injury visualized during fiberoptic nasopharyngoscopy and with the eventual need for endotracheal intubation.

Intrathoracic

Lower trachea. On forced expiration, the pleural pressure surrounding the intrathoracic airway is positive and the flow plateau resulting from an obstruction at this site will be seen on expiration (Fig. 3-1C). The inspiratory loop is not affected. Although $FIF_{50\%}/FEF_{50\%}$ is high and FEV_1 is smaller than FIV_1, as in lower airways

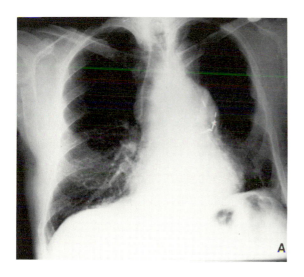

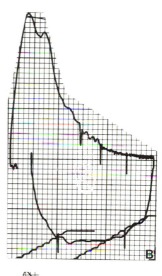

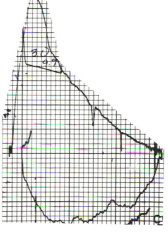

Fig. 3-11. (A) Chest radiograph (PA projection) six months post-left upper lobectomy showing a large mass in the left hilum and mediastinum (recurrent bronchogenic carcinoma) and narrowing of the left main bronchus. (B) F-V loops at the same time as (A) showing well preserved inspiratory and bi-phasic expiratory flow. The first half of the MEFV curve is delivered at high flow, the second half at markedly reduced flow. (C) After two months of radiotherapy, note improvement in the expiratory flow profile. In all graphs, one large division equals one liter of volume and 2 L/sec of flow.

obstruction (including CAO), the configuration of the MEVF curve is different since flows at high lung volume, including peak flow, are primarily affected.

Localized, noncircumferential tumors are the main cause of variable intrathoracic obstruction; tracheomalacia and polychondritis have also been described.

Main bronchus. An obstruction of a main bronchus may produce a biphasic MEVF curve. This results from superimposition of a normal curve from the contralateral lung on an obstructed curve from the lung whose bronchus is blocked. Initial flows are of good amplitude; these are followed by the remaining FVC delivered at low flow.[14,15] This is illustrated in Figure 3-11B. Such a curve may be difficult to differentiate from the curve of airways obstruction, but will normalize if the tumor responds to surgery, radiation, or chemotherapy.

A biphasic curve has also been described[14] in patients with combined restrictive-obstructive impairment; the VC is generally smaller than in unilateral bronchial obstruction. Combined impairment is discussed in Chapter 10.

In exceptional cases, narrowing of both main bronchi may so reduce cross-sectional area of the airway as to simulate more proximal fixed obstruction (see Case Presentation 3-2, above).

COEXISTING LOWER AIRWAYS OBSTRUCTION

Clinicians are aware that many of the factors bringing about UAO (e.g., tracheal intubation for CAO) are associated with lower airways obstruction as well. Since UAO affects inspiratory flow and/or expiratory flow at high lung volume, the effort-independent portion of the MEFV curve is not generally altered and will provide evidence of lower airways obstruction if it is present.

Masking of Lower Airways Obstruction in the Presence of UAO

This may take place with severe fixed UAO in which both loops of the F-V curve are uniformly flattened at all lung volumes.

Masking of UAO in the Presence of Lower Airways Obstruction

Lower airways obstruction may mask variable extrathoracic obstruction by rendering the $FIF_{50\%}/FEF_{50\%}$ ratio meaningless. Inspiratory flow can be markedly decreased and the ratio will still be normal (greater than unity).

References

1. Miller RD, Hyatt RE. Obstructing lesions of the larynx and trachea: Clinical and physiologic characteristics. Mayo Clin Proc 44:145–161, 1969

2. Miller RD, Hyatt RE. Evaluation of obstructing lesions of the trachea and larynx by flow-volume loops. Am Rev Respir Dis 108:475–481, 1973

3. Deckert RE, Burgher LW. Serial flow-volume loops as an aid to management of primary oat cell carcinoma of the trachea. Chest 73:560–561, 1978

4. Miller A, Brown LK, Teirstein AS. Stenosis of main bronchi mimicking fixed upper airway obstruction in sarcoidosis. Chest 88:244–248, 1985

5. Gamsu G, Borson DB, Webb WR, et al. Structure and function in tracheal stenosis. Am Rev Respir Dis 121:519-531, 1980

6. Bergeron D, Cormier Y, Desmeules M. Tracheobronchopathia osteochondroplastica. Am Rev Respir Dis 114:803–806, 1976

7. Lundgren R, Stjernberg NL. Tracheobronchopathia osteochondoplastica. A clinical and spirometric study. Chest 80:706–709, 1981

8. Cormier Y, Kashima H, Summer W, et al. Airflow in unilateral vocal cord paralysis before and after Teflon injection. Thorax 33:57–61, 1978

9. Christopher KL, Wood RP II, Eckert C, et al. Vocal cord dysfunction presenting as asthma. N Engl J Med 308:1566–1570, 1983

10. Collett PW, Brancatisano T, Engel LA. Spasmodic croup in the adult. Am Rev Respir Dis 127:500–504, 1983

11. Haponik EF, Bleecker ER, Allen RP, et al. Abnormal inspiratory flow-volume curves in patients with sleep-disordered breathing. Am Rev Respir Dis 124:571–574, 1981

12. Sanders MH, Martin RJ, Pennock BE, et al. The detection of sleep apnea in the awake patient. The "Saw-Tooth" sign. JAMA 245:2414–2418, 1981

13. Haponik EF, Munster AM, Wise RA, et al. Upper airway function in burn patients. Correlation of flow-volume curves and nasopharyngoscopy. Am Rev Respir Dis 129:251–257, 1984

14. Lord GP. The expiratory flow volume curve in localized airway obstruction. J Maine Med Ass 60:18–20, 1969

15. Lord GP, Gazioglu K, Kaltreider N. The maximum expiratory flow-volume in the evaluation of patients with lung disease. A comparative study with standard pulmonary function tests. Amer J Med 46:72–79, 1969

4

Maximum Voluntary Ventilation

Albert Miller

Definition
Applications
  As an Integrated Measurement of the Ventilatory Process
  In Interstitial Lung Disease
    Air Velocity Index
  In Obstructive Airways Disease
    "Indirect" MVV
  Dynamic Air Trapping
  In Upper Airways Obstruction
  In Chest Bellows Impairments
  To Evaluate Respiratory Muscle Performance
    Effects of Airways Conductance versus Muscle Performance on MVV
    Strength versus Endurance: Maximum Sustained Ventilation
  Evaluation of Respiratory Drive
  Surgical Evaluation
  Disability Evaluation

DEFINITION

The maximum voluntary ventilation (MVV) is the volume of air that a subject can breathe upon repetitive maximal voluntary effort.[1,2] Although the time of the

PULMONARY FUNCTION TESTS: A   ISBN 0-8089-1764-4   Copyright © 1987 by Grune & Stratton
GUIDE FOR THE STUDENT AND HOUSE OFFICER   All rights of reproduction in any form reserved.

test is 10–15 seconds, the result is expressed in L/min. The subject is allowed to select the respiratory rate that will produce the greatest ventilation. There is little difference in normal subjects when different respiratory rates between 60 and 120 per minute are selected.

APPLICATIONS

As an Integrated Measurement of the Ventilatory Process

The greatest value of the MVV is its *nonspecificity,* that it reflects the effects on ventilation whether the disease process is in the neuromuscular apparatus, chest cage or airways. The test measures ventilation as an integrated process involving many systems. Gaensler and Wright[3] expressed this well in 1966:

Performance of this test . . . is affected by the integrity of the respiratory bellows as a whole including such factors as respiratory muscle blood supply, fatigue, and progressive trapping of air. Because of this, the [MVV] . . . correlates more closely with subjective dyspnea than does any other [readily available, easily performed] test.

Aldrich et al[4] quantified the relative contributions of airways conductance and respiratory muscle strength (estimated from maximal inspiratory and expiratory pressures) to MVV. In normal and CAO subjects, MVV correlated best with G_{aw}; in patients with ILD, MVV correlated with respiratory muscle strength.

In Interstitial Lung Disease

Air Velocity Index

The MVV is generally not reduced in ILD until the disease is far advanced, in which case the reduction is less than that in lung volumes or gas exchange. This is reflected by the old-fashioned *Air Velocity Index:*

Equation 4-1

$$\text{Air Velocity Index} = \frac{\text{Percent predicted MVV}}{\text{Percent predicted VC}}$$

This index is far above unity in ILD.

When a well-performed MVV is decreased in a patient with ILD, it suggests additional factors, such as airways obstruction (in chronic fibrotic sarcoidosis or complicated pneumoconiosis), respiratory muscle involvement (in dermatomyositis

---

*From Gaensler EA, Wright GW. Evaluation of respiratory impairment. Arch Environ Health 12:155, 1966, with permission.

or polymyositis), fibrothorax (secondary to fibrous pleurisy in patients with asbestosis) or upper airway obstruction (following intubation or due to laryngeal involvement as in sarcoidosis).

In Obstructive Airways Disease

"Indirect" MVV

In patients with obstructive impairment, the MVV is reduced in proportion to the FEV_1 and may be "predicted" from the FEV_1 by multiplying by a factor of 35–40.[3] Some patients who cannot perform the forced expiratory maneuver find it more natural to perform the rhythmic MVV. If an adequate FEV_1 cannot be obtained from such a patient, a decrease in the hoary air velocity index helps quantitate the degree of airflow obstruction.

Since the MVV is performed above or near the FRC, it is not decreased in patients with small airways disease. This is as expected from the preserved FEV_1 in these patients.

Dynamic Air Trapping

When tidal breathing is recorded at rest and during the MVV, dynamic air trapping is apparent as a *progressive* increase in end-expiratory position, as illustrated in Figure 4-1. The final increase in FRC may be as large as 2L. Concomitant with the increase in lung volume at which tidal breathing takes place, the tidal volume is usually reduced (sometimes to values below 200 cc). Patients with severe emphysema occasionally have a *smaller* ventilatory volume during MVV than during rest. Even if overall ventilation does not fall in such patients, alveolar ventilation may decrease as the smaller tidal volumes simply move air back and forth within the anatomic dead space.

In Upper Airways Obstruction

The MVV is characteristically reduced in UAO, which is an example of disproportionate decrease in MVV compared with FEV_1. The ratio of MVV to FEV_1 was 19.5 in patients with UAO versus 41.0 in normals, 44.0 in ILD, 39.4 in CAO, and 40.6 in asthma.[5]

In Chest Bellows Impairments

Of the large number of variables mentioned earlier in this section that affect the MVV, many relate to the innervation, strength, blood supply, and mechanical advantage of the respiratory muscles and to the expansibility of the rib cage. The MVV is reduced in patients with spinal cord, phrenic nerve or respiratory muscle

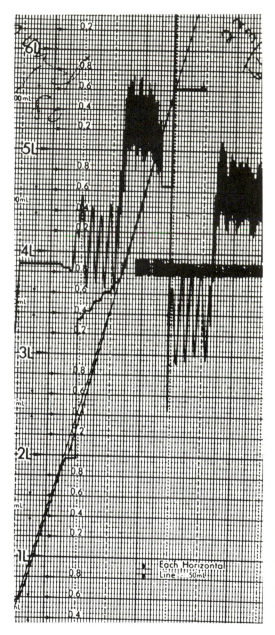

Fig. 4-1. Repeat MVVs performed by a 40-year-old man with generalized tuberculous bronchiectasis and CAO. The tests were identical (73 L/min). Both tidal volume tracings show dynamic air trapping, a stepwise increase in FRC with each breath; the difference in FRC between resting and maximum ventilation is ca. 1550 cc.

involvement; skeletal deformities of the thorax, such as kyphoscoliosis; fibrothorax; obesity and ascites.

Since lung volumes in these conditions may be similar to those seen in ILD, the MVV helps distinguish between types of restrictive impairment. (Restrictive impairments, including chest bellows and neuromuscular, are discussed more fully in Chapter 10.)

To Evaluate Respiratory Muscle Performance

Effects of Airways Conductance versus Muscle Performance on MVV

In the absence of airways obstruction, MVV is a good index of respiratory muscle performance. The ratio of MVV to FEV_1 is decreased in the presence of neuromuscular disease but not to the extent seen in UAO.[5] In the presence of airways obstruction, airways conductance can be taken into account by the following relationship[4]:

Equation 4-2

$$MVV \text{ (percent predicted)} = 353 \, SG_{AW} + 11.5$$

Strength versus Endurance: Maximum Sustained Ventilation

Respiratory muscle performance can be considered as two properties. (1) Strength, assessed by the maximum static pressures developed at the mouth during inspiration and expiration. The MVV is significantly related to these pressures. (2) Endurance, assessed by the capacity for sustaining high levels of ventilation. A measurement of endurance is the maximum sustained ventilation (MSV), the maximum ventilation that can be sustained for 10–15 minutes. The MSV is a relatively constant fraction of the MVV in normal subjects (80 percent[6,7]) and in patients with CAO (50 percent[8]).

It has been pointed out that whereas 100 percent of the MVV can be sustained for less than a minute, 5 percent can be sustained for a lifetime. Energy supply to respiratory muscles may be considered adequate to sustain ventilation at about 55 percent of the MVV in normal subjects.[9] Thus, while MVV is limited by mechanical factors, sustained hyperventilation is limited by the aerobic capacity of the respiratory muscles.[10]

Evaluation of Respiratory Drive

Since the MVV is a test of overall ventilatory function from transmission of the neural impulse to movement of air through the large airways, the observation that it is normal in a patient with ventilatory failure helps eliminate disease at these (and intervening) sites and to establish the diagnosis of primary hypoventilation. That hyperventilation can be achieved normally on volition (and can correct the abnormal blood gases which are present) helps place the lesion at the site where automatic ventilation is controlled.

Surgical Evaluation

The MVV, again because it reflects a large number of important physiologic factors, is a useful parameter in assessing respiratory reserve intraoperatively and postoperatively (see Chapter 13).

Disability Evaluation

To expand Gaensler's 1966 statement, in the opening paragraph of this section on applications, "The MBC (maximum breathing capacity is an older term for MVV) and *its relation to ventilatory requirement* (dyspnea index) correlates more closely with subjective dyspnea [and therefore with respiratory disability] than does any other [readily available] test."[3] The relationship of the MVV to the ventilatory requirement (minute ventilation at rest or on exercise) has been called the "dyspnea index" or "breathing reserve ratio (see chapter 14)."

References

1. Hermannsen J. Untersuchungen uber die maximale ventilationsgrosse (Atem-grenzwert). Z Exp Med 90:130, 1933
2. Warring FC. Ventilatory function. Experiences with a simple practical procedure for its evaluation in patients with pulmonary tuberculosis. Am Rev Tuberc 51:432–454, 1945
3. Gaensler EA, Wright GW. Evaluation of respiratory impairment. Arch Environ Health 12:146–189, 1966
4. Aldrich TK, Arora NS, Rochester DF. The influence of airway obstruction and respiratory muscle strength on maximal voluntary ventilation in lung disease. Am Rev Respir Dis 126:195–199, 1982
5. Owens GR, Murphy DMF. Spirometric diagnosis of upper airway obstruction. Arch Intern Med 143:1331–1334, 1983
6. Shephard RJ. The maximum sustained voluntary ventilation in exercise. Clin Sci 32:167–176, 1967
7. Leith DL, Bradley M. Ventilatory muscle strength and endurance training. J Appl Physiol 41:508–516, 1976
8. Rochester DF, Arora NS, Braun NMT, et al. The respiratory muscles in COPD. Bull Eur Physiopath Resp 15:951–975, 1978
9. Tenney SM, Reese RE. The ability to sustain great breathing efforts. Resp Physiol 5:187–201, 1968
10. Roussos C, Fixley M, Gross D, et al. Fatigue of inspiratory muscles and their synergic behavior. J Appl Physiol 46:897–904, 1979

5

Full Lung Volumes: Functional Residual Capacity, Residual Volume and Total Lung Capacity

Lee K. Brown
and Albert Miller

Methods of Measurement
    Dilutional
      "Wash-in"
      "Wash-out"
    Body Plethysmography
    Radiographic
Application

The VC and FEV_1 are *ventilable* lung volumes, directly measurable by a spirometer during a specific breathing maneuver. The volume of air remaining at the end of a forced expiration or *residual volume* (RV) cannot be measured directly, nor can the other *static lung capacities which include the RV;* these can be measured using the methods discussed below. In actual practice, the functional residual capacity (FRC), or volume at the end of a normal expiration, is measured because it is more reproducible since it is the lung volume at which the respiratory muscles are at rest and the outward retraction of the rib cage is balanced by the inward elastic recoil of the lungs. The ERV is then subtracted from the FRC to obtain the RV. The addition of appropriate directly measured lung volumes to the FRC (or RV) provides the total lung capacity (TLC):

Equation 5-1

$$FRC - ERV = RV$$
$$FRC + \text{Insp. Capacity} = TLC$$
$$RV + VC = TLC$$

METHODS OF MEASUREMENT

Dilutional

"Wash-in"

The patient breathes an insoluble foreign gas (eg, Helium) from a reservoir of known volume and size, thus diluting its concentration by the volume of his lungs (Fig. 5-1). Since amount of He (volume × concentration) does not change and initial volume and concentration are known while final concentration is measured, the only remaining unknown, final volume, can be easily calculated:

Equation 5-2

$$V_{FRC} = \frac{V_{APPARATUS} \times (C_{INIT} - C_{FINAL})}{C_{FINAL}}$$

"Wash-out"

A gas "resident" in the lungs (N_2) is "washed out" by breathing 100 percent O_2 until it reaches negligible concentration (1–2 percent) (Fig. 5-2). The volume and N_2 concentration of all the expired gas are measured; the initial N_2 concentration in the lungs is known (atmospheric):

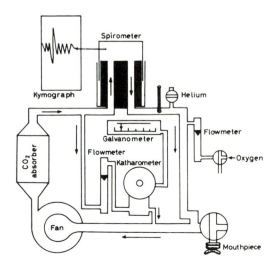

Fig. 5-1. Apparatus for the measurement of FRC by Helium dilution. The flowmeter, katharometer, and galvanometer together comprise the Helium analyzer. [From Cotes JE. Lung Function. Oxford, Blackwell, 1979, p 112, with permission.]

Fig. 5-2. Apparatus for the measurement of FRC by Nitrogen washout. Taps 1 and 2 are provided so that the subject may be switched between the small spirometer circuit and the N_2 washout circuit. When turned to the spirometer circuit, observation of tidal breathing allows correct switching to the washout circuit at FRC. [From Jalowayski AA, Dawson A. Measurement of lung volume: The multiple breath Nitrogen method, in Clausen JL, Pulmonary Function Testing Guidelines and Controversies, New York, Academic Press, 1982, p 117, with permission.]

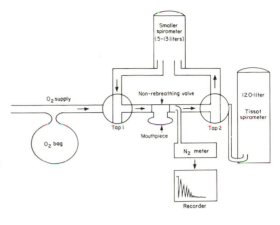

Equation 5-3

$$V_{FRC} = \frac{V_{EXP} \times C_{EXP}}{0.79 - C_{ALV \text{ (FINAL)}}}$$

Both the wash-in and wash-out shown are *multiple breath dilutions* in which the subject breathes until he reaches a constant gas concentration. Each may also be done as a *single breath dilution,* the wash-in as part of the D_LCO_{SB} (Chapter 7) and the wash-out as part of the SB N_2 test (Chapter 6). Although results of MB and SB methods may be comparable in subjects with normal lungs or pure ILD, SB values are unpredictably reduced when airways obstruction leads to air trapping. They are therefore not advised for clinical purposes.

Body Plethysmography

This method is an application of Boyle's Law. It states that in a closed system at constant temperature, the product of pressure and volume within the system remains constant:

Equation 5-4

$$P_1V_1 = P_2V_2$$

Within a body plethysmograph or "body box" (Fig. 5-3), the lungs and upper airways are converted into a closed system by occluding the subject's nose and (briefly!) occluding the mouthpiece. The subject's panting respiratory efforts against the occluded airway change intrathoracic pressure and volume (thoracic gas

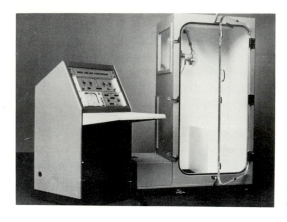

Fig. 5-3. A commercially-manufactured pressure (constant volume) body plethysmograph. [Courtesy of Gould Inc, Dayton, Ohio.]

is rarified as inhalation is attempted; thoracic pressure decreases, and volume increases; Fig. 5-4).

One such inspiratory attempt, when applied to Equation 5-4, yields:

Equation 5-5

$$P_{FRC}V_{FRC} = (P_{FRC} - \Delta P)(V_{FRC} + \Delta V)$$

P_{FRC} = Alveolar pressure = atmospheric pressure (under conditions of zero flow when the airway is occluded) at FRC

V_{FRC} = lung volume at FRC

ΔP = the small decrease in alveolar pressure that occurs with the inspiratory effort

Δv = the small increase in lung volume that occurs with the inspiratory effort

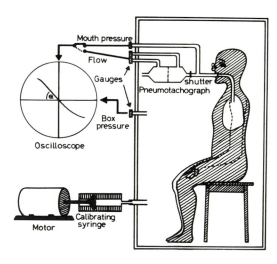

Fig. 5-4. Configuration of a pressure (constant volume) body plethysmograph. [From Cotes JE. Lung Function. Oxford, Blackwell, 1979, p 116, with permission.]

If we solve this equation for V_{FRC}, we obtain:

Equation 5-6

$$V_{FRC} = \frac{\Delta V}{\Delta P} (P_{FRC} - \Delta P)$$

Finally, we may assume that $P_{FRC} - \Delta P = P_{FRC}$, since the magnitude of ΔP is very small compared with P_{FRC}. Substituting, we arrive at:

Equation 5-7

$$V_{FRC} = \frac{\Delta V}{\Delta P} (P_{FRC})$$

Where ΔP is obtained from the change in mouth pressure against the occluded valve and ΔV from the change in pressure in the plethysmograph as air in the box is compressed by an increase in lung volume.

Both plethysmography and multiple breath-dilution are accurate and acceptable for clinical testing. Plethysmography measures the volume of all air containing spaces within the thorax (*thoracic gas volume*). Occasionally, a noncommunicating bulla (or air in a dilated esophagus in a patient with achalasia) will result in a difference between the two methods. This difference is called the *volume of trapped gas*.

The availability of a body plethysmograph allows airways resistance, R_{aw}, or its reciprocal, airways conductance, G_{aw}, to be measured. For most clinical purposes, these measurements do not add to the information obtained from the FEV_1 and flow rates.

Radiographic

The TLC can be approximated from standard posteroanterior and lateral chest radiographs using either planimetry (excluding the heart and mediastinum)[1] or a series of measurements that treat each hemithorax as a stack of ellipsoids of varying size.[2,3] Differences between radiographic and plethysmographic values have been reported[4] and the former are best used for epidemiologic surveys rather than clinical testing.

APPLICATION

Full lung volumes are clinically useful for classifying restrictive impairments, for confirming small airways obstruction (RV is frequently increased) and for quantitating the degree of air trapping in overt airways obstruction. Changes in chest wall elastic recoil will change the FRC in the same direction in ankylosing spondylitis (increased) and Klinefelter's syndrome (decreased). The major application of full lung volumes is in interpreting a decrease in FVC in the presence of airways obstruction: Is the decrease secondary to air trapping (elevated FRC and RV) or an additional restrictive process such as interstitial or pleural fibrosis (FRC, TLC and RV are not increased and may be reduced). These matters are discussed in detail in Chapter 10.

References

1. Harris TR, Pratt PC, Kilburn KH. Total lung capacity measured by roentgenograms. Am J Med 50:756–763, 1971
2. Lloyd HM, String ST, DuBois AB. Radiographic and plethysmographic determination of total lung capacity. Radiology 86:7–14, 1966
3. Ferris BG, Speizer FE, Bishop YMM, et al. Spirometry for an epidemiologic study: Deriving optimum summary statistics for each subject. Bull Physiopathol Resp 14:145–155, 1978
4. Barrett WA, Clayton PD, Lambson CR, et al. Computerized roentgenographic determination of total lung capacity. Am Rev Respir Dis 113:239–244, 1976

6

Distribution of Ventilation, Closing Volume, and Closing Capacity: The Single Breath Nitrogen Washout

E. Neil Schachter

BACKGROUND: THE INHOMOGENEITY OF VENTILATION

The mechanisms that explain the inequalities of ventilation have been grouped under the headings of regional or parallel ventilation differences, and series ventilation effects.

Parallel differences in ventilation relate to gravitational effects, which impose regional variations in the dimensions of the lung; differences in airway length, inequalities of lung tissue compliance, differences in the forces applied to lung tissue regionally, and variations in local airway resistance.

PULMONARY FUNCTION TESTS: A   ISBN 0-8089-1764-4   Copyright © 1987 by Grune & Stratton
GUIDE FOR THE STUDENT AND HOUSE OFFICER   All rights of reproduction in any form reserved.

Series ventilation inequalities refer primarily to redistribution of gases in the terminal airways by diffusion. Under such a heading comes the concept of stratification, which suggests that once gas reaches the terminal units, mainly as a result of convective transport, local diffusion then contributes to inhomogeneity. Differences in time constants of terminal airways may also contribute to inhomogeneity. Another mechanism for redistribution of gas in the small lung units may be collateral ventilation from one alveolar space to another, through the pores of Kohn and the canals of Lambert.

The study of gas distribution in the lung has led to the characterization of two properties of the gas exchange system: first, its size, typified by such measurements as the FRC, RV, and TLC and second, its ability to distribute ventilation, typified by measurements of the anatomic dead space, the closing volume, and the slope of the alveolar phase, all of which are obtained from the single breath N_2 washout curve, the most widely employed technique to assess distribution of ventilation.

THE SINGLE BREATH N_2 WASHOUT

The Four Phases of the Washout Curve

This technique involves the washout of nitrogen from the lungs by a single breath of 100 percent O_2. If one measures the concentration of exhaled nitrogen as a function of exhaled volume, one appreciates four phases of the washout curve as illustrated in Figure 6-1. In phase I, dead space gas containing no nitrogen is exhaled. During phase II the interface gas between dead space and alveolar air is exhaled. The slope of phase II (in contrast to a "step") indicates the dynamic distribution of gas in the two compartments. Phase III of the SB curve has a much shallower slope than Phase II. The gas now analyzed is representative of relatively "even" emptying of alveolar spaces. The slope of this phase, which is called the *alveolar plateau*, is proportional to the inhomogeneity of alveolar emptying, which

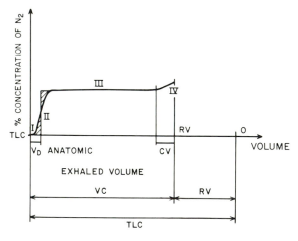

Fig. 6-1. Four phases of the single breath nitrogen washout curve. [From Ruppel G. Manual of Pulmonary Function Testing. St. Louis, C. V. Mosby, 1982, p 51, with permission.]

is accentuated by various disease processes. Phase IV, when it occurs, marks an end of the relatively uniform emptying of alveolar gas and a predominance of gas from the less gravity dependent portion of the lung, or in the case of disease, from regions with a greater time constant. The volume of this last phase has been termed the closing volume, discussed below.

Closing Volume and Closing Capacity

In 1972, McCarthy et al[1] suggested that phase IV might be related to the newly emerging concept of small airways disease. They termed *closing volume* (CV) the volume above residual volume at which the gravity dependent lung zones cease to ventilate as demonstrated by SB washout curves. *Closing capacity* (CC) is simply the absolute lung volume at which "closing" begins.

Equation 6-1

$$CC = CV + RV \text{ (Residual Volume)}$$

Closing volume is standardized against the patient's own VC whereas closing capacity is standardized against his TLC. Since the latter measurement may itself be sensitive to gas trapping, there may be some advantage in using CC rather than CV in assessing mild airways disease.

McCarthy[1] calculated a simple linear regression for CV with age in healthy nonsmokers:

Equation 6-2

$$\text{Closing Volume (as a percentage of VC)} = 1.9 + 0.36 \times \text{age}$$

Smokers had a high prevalence of abnormal values. Twenty years later, the consensus regarding the SB N_2 tests is that although interesting correlations among them, the FEV_1, and other indices of small airways obstruction (flows at low lung volumes, frequency dependence of dynamic compliance, density dependence of flows using 80 percent He-20 percent O_2) have been reported in smokers and in subjects with various diseases or exposures, the clinical usefulness of "small airways tests" remains uncertain.

That airways actually close at low lung volumes in gravity-dependent segments of the lung was confirmed by Hughes et al.[2] His group studied the morphologic changes by means of bronchography and histologic sectioning of rapidly frozen lung.

References

1. McCarthy DS, Spencer R, Greene R, et al. Measurement of "closing volume" as a simple and sensitive test for early detection of small airway disease. Am J Med 52:747–753, 1972
2. Hughes JMB, Rosenzweig DY, Kivitz PB. Site of airway closure in excised dog lungs: Histologic demonstration. J Appl Physiol 29:340–344, 1970

7

Diffusing Capacity (Transfer Factor) for Carbon Monoxide

Albert Miller

Definition
Single Breath Diffusing Capacity for CO (D_LCO_{SB})
  Method
  Calculation
  Physiologic Factors Influencing Results
    Age
    Body Position
    Lung Volume
    Exercise
    Blood Volume and Heart Failure
    Cigarette Smoking and Increase in Venous Carboxyhemoglobin
    Hemoglobin Concentration
    Pregnancy
Clinical Applications
  Interstitial Lung Disease
    Early Diagnosis
    Following the Course of Disease
    Disability Evaluation
    Separation of Interstitial From Pleural Fibrosis
  Chronic Airways Obstruction
    The Diagnosis of Emphysema
    Correlation with Hypoxemia

PULMONARY FUNCTION TESTS: A   ISBN 0-8089-1764-4   Copyright © 1987 by Grune & Stratton
GUIDE FOR THE STUDENT AND HOUSE OFFICER   All rights of reproduction in any form reserved.

Pulmonary Vascular Disease
Increased D_LCO_{SB} and D_LCO/V_A
   Erythrocytosis
   Increased Pulmonary Blood Volume
   Asthma
   Obesity
   Pulmonary Hemorrhage

The diffusing capacity is the only noninvasive, readily available test that provides information on the gas exchange function of the lungs as opposed to their mechanical properties. It therefore provides information that is unavailable by other means, eg, the diffusing capacity of the lungs (D_L) is often reduced when spirometry, lung volumes, and clinical and radiographic examinations are normal. Two gases can be used to measure D_L, namely O_2 and CO. Methods based on O_2 are complicated and require inhalation of high and low concentrations. In clinical testing, only CO methods are used.

DEFINITION

The D_L may be considered a conductance, G or the reciprocal of a resistance, R. It measures the flow, F, of the gas (O_2 or CO) from a region of higher pressure, (the alveoli), to a region of lower pressure (the pulmonary capillary blood), ΔP across a combined resistance, R, which is offered by the alveolar capillary membrane and the chemical reaction of the gas with hemoglobin:

Equation 7-1

$$\text{In general, } R = \frac{\Delta P}{F}, \text{ and } G = \frac{F}{\Delta P}$$

Equation 7-2

$$\text{Specifically, } D_L \text{ (CO or } O_2) = \frac{\text{Uptake, cc/min}}{\Delta PCO^* \text{ or } \Delta PO_2, \text{ mm Hg}}$$

In order for a gas to reflect the properties of the alveolar-capillary membrane, its uptake must be limited by the resistance across this interface, rather than by the pulmonary blood flow. The uptake of almost all soluble gases is limited by pulmonary blood flow, and these (nitrous oxide, acetylene) may be used to measure this parameter. It is only those gases (O_2 and CO) that chemically combine with hemoglobin and therefore have a virtually unlimited "sink" in the pulmonary capillary blood whose transfer is limited by the alveolar-capillary interface. The two major

---

*Pulmonary capillary PCO is negligible and may be discarded.

resistances to diffusion from alveolar air to intracellular hemoglobin therefore reside in the following.

"Alveolar-capillary membrane."   This is about 1μ in thickness and consists of the film of alveolar surface fluid, the attenuated type I alveolar epithelial cell and pulmonary capillary endothelial cell with their basement membranes, and a minimum of connective tissue in between. There is virtually no resistance interposed by the plasma in the pulmonary capillary.

Intracellular stroma and molecular conformation of hemoglobin.   As they enter the red cell, molecules of CO or O_2 combine first with hemoglobin near the outside of the cell. Succeeding molecules of gas must diffuse further into the cell to reach available binding sites. As gas is bound to hemoglobin, local tension decreases, further slowing transfer to binding sites.

The volume of blood within the pulmonary capillaries in normal upright man is roughly the same as the stroke volume of the heart. At a cardiac rate of 75/min, red blood cells require one cardiac cycle (0.75 second) for their transit through the pulmonary capillaries. This transit time is fully adequate for gas exchange at rest.

Because CO, unlike O_2, is not present in appreciable concentrations in the venous return and therefore in pulmonary capillary blood, the pressure gradient from alveolus to pulmonary capillary is determined solely by the alveolar pressure, which can be readily estimated. The 200-times greater affinity of hemoglobin for CO and the small concentrations (0.1–0.3 percent or 1000–3000 ppm) of this gas used in testing ensure that the pulmonary capillary pressure remains negligible.

SINGLE BREATH DIFFUSING CAPACITY FOR CO (D_LCO_{SB})

This is the most widely used, most standardized method for measuring the diffusing capacity. It requires no arterial puncture, is easily performed and quickly repeated and can demonstrate excellent reproducibility. Our discussion of the diffusing capacity will concern the SB method.

Method

The standards for performing and calculating the D_LCO_{SB} that follow conform to the Epidemiology Standardization Project,[1] the 1984 ATS Alta Conference on Standardization of the D_LCO,[2] and other recommendations.[3] The inspirate should contain 0.25–0.35 percent CO, 10 percent He (or another inert gas), and 21 percent O_2 at sea level; the balance is N_2.

The subject expires maximally to RV (through the first port of a 5-way valve, open to room air). The timer for breath holding is set, the valve is turned to the inspiratory gas (the second port) and the patient rapidly inspires to TLC. After

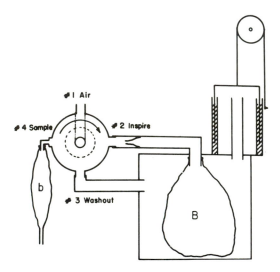

Fig. 7-1. Conventional bag-in-box system for D_LCO_{SB} utilizing a 5-way valve that s turned clockwise either manually or by an automatic sequencer. Positions are: #1, room air, at which the subject expires completely; #2, inspiratory bag (B), which contains the CO-He mixture; inspired volume is measured by a spirometer connected to the box in which the bag is located; #3, dead space washout; this may be into the box, allowing the volume to be measured by the spirometer or into a bag whose volume change is detected by the valve sequencer; #4, alveolar sample bag (b). The volume of this sample can be judged by its distention or measured by placing the bag in a chamber. After collecting the alveolar sample, the remaining expiration is made to room air (#1). The hose from the inspiratory bag B is flushed with test mixture by pressing on the spirometer; rebreathing may be prevented by a valve. [From Gaensler EA, Smith AA, Attachment for automated single breath diffusing capacity measurement. Chest 63:137, 1973, with permission.]

reaching maximum inspiration, the subject holds her breath for the remainder of the 10 second breath-holding time (BHT). She then expires rapidly through the third port sufficient volume to assure that her anatomic dead space has been cleared (750–1000 cc). After the dead space gas has been discarded, an "alveolar" sample of 500–1000 cc is collected for analysis through the fourth port, into a nondiffuseable bag. The apparatus and valve-sequencing of the conventional bag-in-the-box system are shown in Figure 7-1.

Calculation

The equation for D_LCO_{SB} is shown below. Since D_L is reported STPD, the alveolar volume (V_A) calculated from the inspired volume (Vinsp) is converted from ATPS or ATPD by the appropriate factor (Table 2-1). (As measured, Vinsp is

ATPD when inspiration is made from a bag recently filled by a tank of gas or from a demand valve, and ATPS when made from the bell of a water spirometer).

Equation 7-3

$$D_L CO_{SB} = V_A \times \frac{60}{BHT \text{ (sec)} \times P_B - 47 \text{ (Torr)}} \times \ln \frac{CO \text{ insp*} \times He \text{ exp}}{CO \text{ exp} \times He \text{ insp*}}$$

The V_A is calculated from the Vinsp, corrected for the dilution of He in the inspired gas by the RV. This (less the valve dead space) is the single breath TLC (TLC_{SB}) from which the anatomic dead space (150 ml) is subtracted to obtain the V_A:

Equation 7-3a

$$TLC_{SB} = \left\{ Vinsp \text{ (cc)} \times \frac{He \text{ insp*}}{He \text{ exp}} \right\} - Valve \text{ dead space}$$

$$V_A = (TLC_{SB} - Anatomic \text{ dead space}) \times STPD \text{ factor}$$

The He dilution can be measured after breath holding because He, being insoluble, changes negligibly in concentration during this time. The dilution of helium also provides the initial concentration of CO in the alveoli. This is included in Equation 7-3 and is shown here by itself:

Equation 7-3b

$$Initial \text{ alveolar CO concentration} = CO \text{ insp*} \times \frac{He \text{ exp}}{He \text{ insp*}}$$

The final CO concentration is measured directly in the expired gas (CO exp) after the dead space has been cleared.

The determinants of a diffusing capacity, as shown in Equation 7-2, are thus available. The amount (in cc) of CO transferred is calculated from the concentration of alveolar CO at the beginning and at the end of the BHT and from the V_A. The *mean* alveolar CO concentration is integrated from the initial and final values using the natural logarithm (l_n).

The mean capillary ("back") tension of CO can be ignored. If correction is desired (as for heavy smokers or subjects exposed to high levels of atmospheric CO), back tension may be estimated from an "alveolar" sample after breath hold or from CO hemoglobin in the blood. This is subtracted from the initial (Equation 7-3b) and final alveolar CO values.

Because of the need to clear the dead space and to have sufficient expirate for gas analysis, the SB method cannot be used to measure $D_L CO$ in patients with a VC much < 1.5 L.

---

*Inspired concentration may be set at 100.

Physiologic Factors Influencing Results

Age

The D_L falls with age in adults as does alveolar surface area. The decrease for a male 68 inches in height from age 20 years to age 70 years in our Michigan study[4] is 11.45 cc/min/Torr, which is 31 percent of his value at age 20 years.

Body Position

The test is performed in the upright position. Values increase in the supine position because of increased perfusion of upper zones.[5-7]

Lung Volume

Lung volume at TLC is reflected in the equation for D_LCO_{SB}. Many factors that change lung volume will affect the D_L.

The measured D_LCO_{SB} decreased in a nonlinear fashion as the *lung volume at which the breath is held* decreases. A 50 percent decrease in V_A from TLC results in a 40 percent decrease in D_LCO_{SB}.[8]

Exercise

The total capacity of the pulmonary capillary bed is about 200 cc, of which about one-third is used at rest (pulmonary capillary blood volume = 70 cc). With exercise, cardiac output increases and more of the total capacity is used as unopened pulmonary capillaries are recruited. As a result, perfusion matches more perfectly with ventilation and D_LCO increases.

The increase in D_LCO with exercise has been utilized as a clinical test with steady-state methods, which are not discussed in this book. The D_LCO_{SB} can also be measured during and after exercise. Yasukouchi[9] noted a linear increase when D_LCO_{SB} was plotted against work load (in watts) or VO_2. This increase was caused by an increase in capillary volume. The author proposed using the D_L to evaluate pulmonary capillary distensibility.

As cardiac output and pulmonary blood flow increase with exercise, the transit time of a red blood cell in the pulmonary capillary bed decreases from 0.75 to as low as 0.3 second. In normal subjects, this time is still sufficient to allow equilibration for O_2. During exercise in subjects who inhale a low concentration of O_2 or in patients with parenchymal lung disease, blood may leave the pulmonary capillaries before reaching equilibrium with the O_2 in alveolar gas. (Equilibration with CO_2 is much more rapid and seldom becomes a problem.)

Blood Volume and Heart Failure

Increased blood volume (or red blood cell mass) in the lungs may increase the D_L through increased upper zone perfusion and/or recruitment of capillaries. This may occur early in mitral stenosis or left to right shunting while later in the course, when pulmonary vascular resistance is high, D_L is often decreased.[10] When pulmonary capillaries are engorged, there are more red blood cells to take up CO (the effect of which is to increase D_L) but these cells no longer traverse the pulmonary capillary "single file" so that the distance from alveolar gas to the more distant red cells is widened. We have noted in our clinical laboratory that many patients with chronic left ventricular disease (dilated cardiomyopathy) have values for D_LCO_{SB} that are much lower than their values for VC or TLC. This may relate to pulmonary vascular changes or to decrease in cardiac output.

Cigarette Smoking and Increase in Venous Carboxyhemoglobin

All D_LCO measurements are based on the assumption that PCO in the venous (and thus pulmonary capillary) blood is negligible. When venous COHb is elevated, D_L as it is usually measured is underestimated (see below).

Factors that increase COHb: Cigarette smoke. The median COHb level in smokers is 5.0 percent[11]; values of 12 percent are not unusual. The level in nonsmokers is 1.2 percent (corresponding to 7 ppm), two to three times the baseline level of 0.4–0.6 percent brought about by production of CO in metabolism.

External exposure to combustion. Fire fighters, tunnel attendants, and garage workers are exposed to high levels of CO.

However, increased COHb does not explain the roughly 15 percent lower values for D_LCO_{SB} in otherwise normal smokers. We noted differences of 5.4 ml/mm Hg/min for male current smokers, 2.3 for male exsmokers, and 3.6 for female current smokers, and we published prediction equations that account for effects of smoking.[4]

Hemoglobin Concentration

The D_LCO_{SB} is reduced when hemoglobin concentration is reduced. Cotes et al. studied 20 women with iron-deficiency anemia before and after treatment with iron.[12] They arrived at an equation that corrected for differences in Hb concentration from normal. (This was taken to be 14.6 g/100 ml for both sexes.)

Equation 7-4

$$\text{Standardized } D_LCO_{SB} = \text{obs } D_LCO_{SB} \times \frac{10.2* + \text{obs Hb, g/100 ml}}{1.7\dagger \times \text{obs Hb}}$$

This correction is not linear; it increases hyperbolically with the degree of anemia as shown in Table 7-1.

Pregnancy

Milne[14] measured D_LCO_{SB} repeatedly during pregnancy. Values were higher (than postpartum) in the first 3 months (mean ca. 25 cc/min/mm Hg) and fell to a low value at about 25 weeks (mean ca. 21). Adjustments for the lower hemoglobin and alveolar volumes of pregnancy did not fully account for the changes. The

Table 7-1
Correction Factors for Standardized D_LCO_{SB}
in Anemia

Hb	Correction	Correction G Hb below normal*	$\dfrac{obs}{std} \times 100$
12	1.09	1.035	91.7
10	1.19	1.041	ა4.0
8	1.34	1.052	74.6
6	1.59	1.069	62.8

*14.6
Data calculated using Cotes[52] equation.

decrease in D_LCO_{SB} is not explained, especially in view of the increased cardiac output of pregnancy.

Clinical Applications

A useful way to think of D_LCO_{SB} is as an index of the surface area available for gas exchange. It is reduced when the pulmonary capillary network is attenuated by alveolar thinning and disruption (emphysema), obliterated by alveolar inflammation and fibrosis or obstructed by embolism or vasculitis. Thickening of the alveolar-capillary interface accounts for decrease in D_L when edema fluid, hyaline membranes or exudates are present; thickening may play a minor role in parenchymal fibrosis as well. Disease processes involving the surface area, thickness, and diffusing properties of the alveolar capillary membrane need not be paralleled by a loss in alveolar volume (in the example of emphysema, decreased surface area is associated with increased volume), so that D_L/V_A is often decreased. In later stages or with different patterns of fibrosis, loss of lung volume may be more prominent.

In our experience, patients with a pneumonectomy or reduced lung volumes secondary to chest wall or neuromuscular disorders but with normal lungs often have a smaller decrease in D_LCO_{SB} than in V_A and consequently a higher D_L/V_A. A preserved or higher D_L/V_A indicates "entrapped" rather than fibrotic lungs.

Interstitial Lung Disease

Early Diagnosis

Decrease in D_LCO is often the first abnormality in pulmonary function in patients with ILD. Indeed, a decreased D_L may be present when radiographic and clinical examinations are normal.

---

*14.6 × 0.7
†1.0 + 0.7

Normal roentgenogram. Of 44 patients with biopsy-confirmed disease and normal films reported by Epler, McLoud, et al[15], D_LCO_{SB} was abnormal in 73 percent, VC in 57 percent, and TLC in only 16 percent. The authors proposed that a D_LCO_{SB} value less than 50 percent of predicted be an indication for lung biopsy when the chest x-ray is normal and airway obstruction is not demonstrated (so that emphysema is unlikely).

Case Presentation 7-1 is a 37-year-old black woman with shortness of breath on walking 1–2 blocks. She had been found to have systemic lupus erythematosus two years earlier when she presented with pericarditis and was being treated with corticosteriods. Pulmonary function tests (Table 7-2) revealed moderate restrictive impairment with a marked reduction in D_LCO_{SB} and D_L/V_A. The lungs were normal on clinical and radiographic examination (Fig. 7-2A). Four years later, she was unable to walk a half-block or the slightest incline. Physical examination now revealed fine ("cellophane") rales and basal reticular infiltrates were seen on the chest film (Fig. 7-2B).

Normal spirometry. The contribution of D_LCO_{SB} was evaluated in patients with normal lung mechanics (FVC ≥ 80 percent of predicted and FEV_1/FVC ≥ 0.70). Of 794 such patients, 139 or 17.5 percent had an abnormal D_LCO_{SB} (≤ 80

Table 7-2

Case Presentation 7-1, Physiologic Impairment
Preceding Radiographic Abnormality in Systemic
Lupus Erythematosus, 37-Year-Old Black
Female Nonsmoker, 167 cm, 89 kg*

	3/80	7/83
Lung Volumes		
VC (cc)	2170(66%)	1950 (62%)
ERV	900	700
FRC (plet)	1860	1480
TLC	3130(70%)	2730 (63%)
RV	960(80%)	780 (65%)
Spirometry and Flows		
FVC (cc)	2170(66%)	1880 (60%)
FEV_1	1950(75%)	1730 (71%)
FEV_1/FVC	0.90	0.92
$FEF_{25-75\%}$ (L/sec)	3.02(89%)	2.88 (89%)
MVV (L/min)	90(84%)	119 (115%)
D_LCO_{SB} (cc/min/Torr)	9.0(37%)	8.1 (34%)
D_L/V_A	2.79	2.9†(62%)
PaO_2 (rest, Torr)		91
$PaCO_2$ (rest)		38
pH (rest)		7.40
PaO_2 (2 min exercise)		55

*See footnote to Table 1-1, page 7, for a description of predicted
values used for table showing pulmonary function test results.
†Predicted value 4.70.

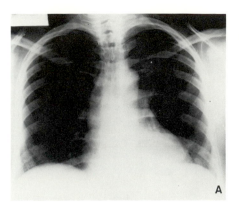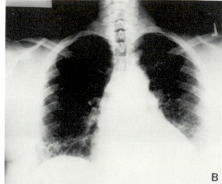

Fig. 7-2. Case Presentation 7-1. Chest radiographs of a dyspneic Hispanic woman with systemic lupus erythematosus. **(A)** in 1980, shows a borderline enlargement of the heart and normal lung fields. **(B)** in 1983, shows well defined reticular infiltrates most pronounced in the lower zones. Pulmonary function tests were abnormal for three years before these radiographic findings were detected.

percent of predicted). In all but one of these, the presence of lung disease was confirmed by radiographic examination or biopsy.[16] (Of the 139, 32 had a normal x-ray and were included in Epler's series cited above.) Gaensler (in Ferris, 1978) concluded that "the D_LCO_{SB} demonstrates significantly impaired gas exchange in one fifth of patients who have no significant defect in mechanics of breathing."[1] This estimate was confirmed by Finnish investigators in 100 consecutive patients with cryptogenic fibrosing alveolitis: the initial FVC was decreased (<80 percent of predicted) in 70; the D_LCO_{SB} was decreased (≤ 75 percent of predicted) in all 97 tested.[17]

The experience in our clinical laboratory has more than confirmed these observations on the usefulness of the D_LCO_{SB}. We have frequently noted diffusion impairment as the only abnormality in patients who complain of shortness of breath and have underlying diseases such as progressive systemic sclerosis or disseminated lupus erythematosus. Involvement of the lungs has been confirmed by biopsy, by radiography either initially or after progression of the disease, or by improvement in D_L along with other evidence of disease upon appropriate therapy.

Sarcoidosis. Marked reduction in D_LCO_{SB} in patients with sarcoidosis who have a normal chest x-ray (stage 0) was illustrated by Figure 1-3 and Table 1-3.

In addition, stage 1 sarcoidosis is a paradigm of ILD with negative radiographic findings in the lungs, since this stage is defined as hilar adenopathy with clear lung fields. In 22 such patients we reported[18], mean D_LCO_{SB} was 72.7 percent of predicted. Twelve patients (55 percent) had values <75 percent of predicted; in contrast, no more than 20 percent had a reduced FVC and/or TLC. The frequency of abnormal D_LCO in stage I sarcoidosis is consistent with the observations that cellular interstitial infiltrates and/or granulomas are almost universally present on lung biopsy even though they are not evident on x-ray.

Opportunistic pulmonary infection in acquired immune deficiency syndrome (AIDS). The D_LCO_{SB} has been valuable in evaluating diffuse opportunistic pulmonary infection in immunocompromised hosts. We found the test frequently to be the only abnormal quickly available finding in dyspneic patients in high risk groups whose opportunistic infections were then demonstrated by fiberoptic bronchoscopy.[19] As our threshold of clinical awareness of AIDS increased, we used the D_LCO_{SB} to evaluate patients for invasive diagnostic procedures who did not have dyspnea or fever, let alone other clinical or radiographic findings. (See Case Presentation 1-2.) Increase in D_L reflects response to treatment of the opportunistic infection.

Following the Course of Disease

The D_LCO_{SB} has been considered an objective evaluator of the course of ILD and the effect of therapy. Prognosis in 100 consecutive patients with nonspecific ILD correlated with the D_LCO_{SB}. Survival was longer when this was ≥ 45 percent of predicted but did not correlate with FVC or histologic appearance.[17] Crystal's group[20,21] emphasized that pulmonary function tests, especially D_LCO_{SB}, reflect structural derangements and particularly loss of alveolar capillary bed. These result from "inactive" fibrosis as well as "active" alveolitis and granuloma formation. Tests of lung function would, therefore, correlate more closely with exercise tolerance and dyspnea than with systemic symptoms like fever or with the activity of the imflammatory process. Nevertheless, associations exist between D_LCO_{SB} and such indices of activity as 67-gallium uptake and the proportion of lymphocytes and T-lymphocytes recovered from bronchoalveolar lavage. Lung function deteriorates when the proportion of T-lymphocytes remains high and is stable when the proportion remains low.

We have reported a correlation between D_L and radiographic stage of sarcoidosis. Contrasted with a mean D_LCO_{SB} 72.7 percent of predicted in stage I, the mean value was 62.0 percent in stage II, in which infiltrates as well as hilar adenopathy are seen on x-ray; 55 percent of the former had a value < 75 percent of predicted contrasted with 92 percent of the latter.[18] Significant hypoxemia ($PaO_2 \leq 69$ Torr) in sarcoidosis is seen only in patients with low D_LCO_{SB}.[22]

The D_LCO_{SB} is useful in evaluating response to therapy in sarcoidosis. We have noted that the increase in D_L is often slower than the improvement in VC and chest x-ray.[23]

This is illustrated by Case Presentation 7-2, a 49-year old white male who presented in September, 1980 with a marked, diffuse reticulonodular infiltrate and no symptoms of which he was aware (Fig. 7-3). Both transbronchial biopsy and a Kveim test were positive for sarcoidosis. Pulmonary function tests are shown in Table 7-3. All lung volumes were reduced. Flows at low lung volume were reduced. The D_LCO_{SB} was half the smoking-specific predicted value. With the initiation of corticosteroid therapy, the patient noted an improve-

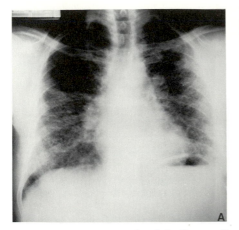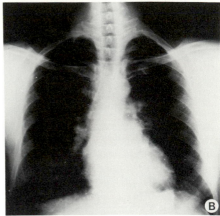

Fig. 7-3. Case Presentation 7-2. Chest radiographs of an "asymptomatic" white man with sarcoidosis. (A) on 9/16/80, shows a profuse reticular-finely nodular infiltrate less apparent in the apices; the hila and paratracheal areas are prominent. (B) on 4/14/82, shows clearing of the infiltrates and borderline lymphadenopathy. Note the increase in lung volume. The patient reported that breathing was much easier and effort tolerance greater.

Table 7-3
Case Presentation 7-2, Response to Corticosteroid Therapy
in Sarcoidosis, 49-Year-Old Male Exsmoker, 175 cm, 75 kg

	9/80	7/81	10/82
Lung Volumes			
VC (cc)	2920 (58%)	4130(83%)	4010(82%)
FRC (plet)	2180	3130	2950
TLC	4210 (55%)	6460(85%)	5610(72%)
RV	1290 (49%)	2330(88%)	1600(58%)
Spirometry and Flows			
FVC (cc)	2920 (58%)	4130(83%)	4010(82%)
FEV_1(L)	2.08 (57%)	3.18(88%)	2.99(81%)
FEV_1/FVC	0.71	0.77	0.75
$FEF_{25-75\%}$ (L/sec)	1.18 (32%)	2.69(75%)	2.23(62%)
MET (sec)	—	0.80	0.90
$FEF_{50\%}$ (L/sec)	2.34	3.66	3.24
$FEF_{75\%}$	0.44	0.74	0.70
R_{aw} (cm H_2O/L/sec)	1.2	—	—
MVV (L/min)	153 (118%)	161(133%)	163(138%)
D_LCO_{SB} (cc/min/Torr)	14.9†(51%)*	17.7(61%)*	23.0(80%)*
PaO_2 (rest, Torr)	74	72	—
PaO_2 (2 min exercise)	67	65	—

*Predicted values are for exsmokers.
†Lower 95 percent confidence limit 20.9.

ment in exercise tolerance, his chest x-ray began to clear and his VC progressively increased. Ten months later, lung volumes were normal but D_LCO_{SB} had improved little. Two years later, lung volumes remained normal and D_L had increased to normal on a small maintenance dose.

Disability Evaluation

As illustrated above, a marked reduction in D_L may be the only readily demonstrable abnormality in patients with a wide variety of interstitial disorders. The American Thoracic Society Committee on Evaluating Respiratory Disability/Impairment[24] following Epler,[25] considers a D_LCO_{SB} value ≤ 50 percent of predicted to be a criterion for disability in ILD irrespective of other findings. Impairment of such degree is likely to limit oxygen transfer at low levels of exercise. This guideline was confirmed by the Boston University Group, who noted that an increase in $\Delta P(A-a)O_2$ on exercise, due primarily to a fall in PaO_2, correlated with the D_LCO_{SB}, being noted when values were below 50–70 percent of predicted.[26] Morrison[27] noted a correlation between D_LCO_{SB} and PaO_2 on step exercise in ILD.

Separation of Interstitial from Pleural Fibrosis

This problem may arise in a patient with asbestosis. A normal or high D_L/V_A suggests that restrictive impairment is primarily pleural.

Chronic Airways Obstruction

The Diagnosis of Emphysema

Chronic bronchitis, chronic asthma, and emphysema show similar physiologic findings of airways obstruction, hyperinflation, and air trapping. Emphysema can be separated from the other causes of CAO by two types of physiologic test. Both reflect the loss of lung tissue that is the essential lesion in emphysema:

A reduction in recoil pressure or an increase in static lung compliance. These measurements require placement of an esophageal balloon.

A reduction in D_L. Gelb[28] examined the lung tissue of 14 patients who underwent resection for localized disease. Of 10 patients with reduced flows, the seven who had reduced D_LCO_{SB} values showed morphologic evidence of emphysema. Morphologic emphysema was not present in the three patients with reduced flows and normal D_LCO_{SB}. More recently, Berend and coworkers[29] confirmed that D_LCO correlated with the degree of emphysema seen morphologically and concluded that it was the most useful test for detecting early emphysema. The relationship between D_LCO_{SB} and morphologic emphysema is shown in Fig. 7-4.

Teculescu[30] noted a similar relationship between D_LCO_{SB} and emphysema as defined clinically and radiographically rather than morphologically. Mean values were 59 percent of predicted in the emphysema group, versus 93 percent in patients

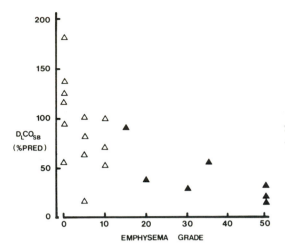

Fig. 7-4. The relationship between D_LCO_{SB} expressed as percent predicted and morphologic grade of emphysema determined from lobectomy specimens. (R = -0.72, p < 0.001). Solid triangles are patients with emphysema. [From Berend N, Woolcock AJ, Marlin GE. Correlation between the function and structure of the lung in smokers. Am Rev Respir Dis 119:700, 1979, with permission.]

with chronic bronchitis. Eleven of 14 emphysema patients had an abnormal D_L compared with only one of 10 with bronchitis.

Correlation with Hypoxemia

The D_LCO_{SB} was found to identify patients with CAO who desaturated on incremental exercise.[31] None of the 20 patients with a D_L >55 percent of predicted desaturated, while 19 of 28 patients ≤55 percent of predicted did so. The frequency and severity of desaturation increased as the D_L fell. The test has been used to identify patients with CAO likely to benefit from O_2 therapy during exercise. (Note the similar correlation of D_L and exercise-induced hypoxemia in ILD, discussed above.)

Pulmonary Vascular Disease

In the pulmonary laboratory, a decrease in D_LCO_{SB} may be the only readily available evidence for multiple pulmonary emboli,[32,33] idiopathic pulmonary hypertension (which is associated with anatomic changes in the small pulmonary arteries),[34] or pulmonary vasculitis. Increase in physiologic dead space is confirmatory. In a recent study[35] of patients who had pulmonary hypertension, five of six with thromboembolism and nine of fifteen with primary pulmonary hypertension had a low D_LCO. This was the only abnormal pulmonary function test in six (of the 14) patients.

Clinically, and even at postmortem examination, pulmonary vasculitis may be present without parenchymal fibrosis in progressive systemic sclerosis.[36] The D_LCO_{SB} is significantly lower in this disease when pulmonary arterial pressure is elevated; a value <43 percent of predicted was the most sensitive finding to detect pulmonary hypertension.[37] The poor correlation between VC and D_L in progressive systemic sclerosis suggests that the interstitial fibrosis and pulmonary vasculitis are separate processes.

Patients with Raynaud's phenomenon experience spasm in vascular beds other than digital, eg, pulmonary, coronary, and cerebral, leading to migraine headaches. (Indeed, Raynaud's phenomenon may occur in primary pulmonary hypertension.) Subjects with primary Raynaud's phenomenon demonstrated a significant decrease in D_LCO_{SB} after a 2 minute immersion of the hands in 15°C water.[38]

Increased D_LCO_{SB} and D_LCO/V_A

Erythrocytosis

See *Blood volume and heart failure, and Hemoglobin concentration*, above.

Increased Pulmonary Blood Volume

This occurs in exercise and in heart failure, discussed above.

Asthma

See *Chronic Airways Obstruction* above.

Obesity

The D_LCO_{SB} and more so, the D_LCO/V_A tend to increase proportionate to the degree of obesity. Of 43 healthy obese patients studied by Ray et al[39], nine (21 percent) had high values for D_L, which the authors postulated were secondary to the increase in pulmonary (and total) blood volume.

Pulmonary Hemorrhage

Several investigators have noted that D_LCO_{SB} (or D_L/V_A) is frequently increased in patients with fresh intraalveolar hemorrhage.[40] The red blood cells in the alveoli provide extra binding sites for CO. Since CO can only combine with intact hemoglobin, an elevated D_LCO_{SB} reflects recent bleeding. Greening and Hughes[41] used serial tests to follow 27 cases, 70 percent of whom had Goodpasture's syndrome. The increase in D_LCO_{SB} was the most sensitive indication of parenchymal hemorrhage; hemoptysis was absent or minimal (in contrast to bronchial hemorrhage) and radiographic changes often lagged by 24 hours.

References

1. Ferris BG (Principal Investigator). Epidemiology standardization project. Am Rev Respir Dis 118, Part 2, 1978
2. American Thoracic Society Alta Conference. Single breath carbon monoxide diffusing capacity (transfer factor). Preliminary recommendations for a standard technique. ATS News 12:2, 6–12, 1986

3. Make B, Miller A, Epler G, et al. Single breath diffusing capacity in the industrial setting. Chest 82:351–356, 1982

4. Miller A, Thornton JC, Warshaw R, et al. Single breath diffusing capacity in a representative sample of the population of Michigan, a large industrial state: Predicted values, lower limits of normal, and frequencies of abnormality by smoking history. Am Rev Respir Dis 127:270–277, 1983

5. Bates DV, Pearce JF. The pulmonary diffusing capacity; a comparison of methods of measurement and a study of the effect of body position. J. Physiol 132:232, 1956

6. Lewis BM, Lin T, Noe FF, et al. The measurement of pulmonary capillary blood volume and pulmonary membrane diffusing capacity in normal subjects: The effects of exercise and position. J Clin Invest 37:1061, 1958

7. Hyland RH, Krastins IRB, Aspin N, et al. Effect of body position on carbon monoxide diffusing capacity in asymptomatic smokers and nonsmokers. Am Rev Respir Dis 117:1045–1053, 1978

8. Cardigan JB, Marks A, Ellicott MF, et al. An analysis of factors affecting the measurement of pulmonary diffusing capacity by the single breath method. J. Clin Invest 40:1495–1514, 1961

9. Yasukouchi A. Uniformity of increase in pulmonary diffusing capacity during submaximal exercise in normal young adults. Industr Health 22:137–151, 1984

10. Burgess JH. Pulmonary diffusing capacity in disorders of the pulmonary circulation. Chest 49:541–550, 1974

11. Stewart RD, Baretta ED, Platte LR. Carboxyhemoglobin levels in American blood donors. JAMA 229:1187–1196, 1974

12. Cotes JE, Dabbs JM, Elwood PC, et al. Iron deficiency anemia: Its effect on transfer factor for the lung and ventilation and cardiac frequency during submaximal exercise. Clin Sci 49:325–335, 1972

13. Clark EH, Woods RL, Hughes JMB. Effect of blood transfusion on the carbon monoxide transfer factor of the lung in man. Clin Sci Mol Med 54:627–631, 1978

14. Milne JA, Mills RJ, Coutts JRT, et al. The effect of human pregnancy on the pulmonary transfer factor for carbon monoxide as measured by the single-breath method. Clin Sci Mol Med 53:271–276, 1977

15. Epler GR, McLoud TC, Gaensler EA, et al. Normal chest roentgenograms in chronic diffuse infiltrative lung disease. N Engl J Med 298:934–939, 1978

16. Lyons LD, Morrissey WL, Waddell WC, et al. Single breath diffusing capacity for screening. Am Rev Respir Dis 115:350A, 1977

17. Tukianen P, Taskinen E, Holsti P, et al. Prognosis of cryptogenic fibrosing alveolitis. Thorax 38:349–355, 1983

18. Miller A, Chuang M, Teirstein AS, et al. Pulmonary function in stages I and II pulmonary sarcoidosis. Ann NY Acad Sci 278:292–300, 1976

19. Tow TWY, Miller A, Brown LK, et al. $D_L CO_{SB}$ in screening for *Pneumocystis carinii pneumonia* (PCP) in patients with acquired immunodeficiency syndrome (AIDS). Am Rev Respir Dis 129:55, 1984

20. Crystal RG, Roberts WC, Hunninghake GW, et al. Pulmonary sarcoidosis: A disease characterized and perpetuated by activated lung T-lymphocytes. Ann Intern Med 94:73–94, 1981

21. Line RB, Hunninghake GW, Keogh BA, et al. Gallium[-67] scanning to stage the alveolitis of sarcoidosis: Correlation with clinical studies, pulmonary function studies and bronchoalveolar lavage. Am Rev Respir Dis 123:440–446, 1981

22. Matthews JI, Hooper RG. Exercise testing in pulmonary sarcoidosis. Chest 83:75–81, 1983

23. Miller A, Teirstein AS, Chuang MT. The sequence of physiologic changes in pulmonary sarcoidosis: Correlation with radiographic stages and response to therapy. Mt. Sinai J Med 44:852–865, 1977

24. American Thoracic Society. Evaluation of impairment/disability secondary to respiratory disease. Am Rev Respir Dis 126:945–951, 1982

25. Epler GR, Saber FA, Gaensler EA. Determination of severe impairment (disability) in interstitial lung disease. Am Rev Respir Dis 121:647–659, 1980

26. Risk C, Epler GR, Gaensler EA. Exercise alveolar-arterial oxygen pressure difference in interstitial lung disease. Chest 85:69–74, 1984

27. Morrison D, Kory R, Goldman A. The step exercise test in interstitial lung disease. Chest 74:345, 1978

28. Gelb AF, Gold WM, Wright RR. Physiologic diagnosis of subclinical emphysema. Am Rev Resp Dis 107:50–63, 1973

29. Berend N, Woolcock AJ, Marlin GE. Correlation between the function and structure of the lung in smokers. Am Rev Respir Dis 119:695–705, 1979

30. Teculescu DB, Stanescu DC. Lung diffusing capacity. Normal values in male smokers and nonsmokers using the breath-holding technique. Scan J Resp Dis 51:137–149, 1970

31. Owens GR, Rogers RM, Pennock BE, et al. The diffusing capacity as a predictor of arterial oxygen desaturation during exercise in patients with chronic obstructive pulmonary disease. N Engl J Med 310:1218–1221, 1984

32. Jones NL, Goodwin JF. Respiratory function in pulmonary thromboembolic disorders. Br Med J 1:14, 1965

33. Nadel JA, Gold WM, Burgess JH. Early diagnosis of chronic pulmonary vascular obstruction: Value of pulmonary function tests. Am J Med 44:16–25, 1968

34. Fuster V, Steele PM, Edwards WD, et al. Primary pulmonary hypertension: Natural history and the importance of thrombosis. Circulation 70:580–587, 1984

35. D'Alonzo GE, Bower JS, Dantzker DR. Differentiation of patients with primary and thromboembolic pulmonary hypertension. Chest 85:457–461, 1984

36. Young RH, Mark GJ. Pulmonary vascular changes in scleroderma. Am J Med 64:998–1004, 1978

37. Ungerer RG, Tashkin DP, Furst D, et al. Pulmonary artery hypertension in progressive systemic sclerosis. Am J Med 75:65–74, 1983

38. Fahey PJ, Utell MJ, Condemi JJ, et al. Raynaud's phenomenon of the lung. Am J Med 76:263–269, 1984

39. Ray CS, Sue DY, Bray G, et al. Effects of obesity on respiratory function. Am Rev Respir Dis 128:501–506, 1983

40. Ewan PW, Jones HA, Rhodes GG, et al. Detection of intrapulmonary hemorrhage with carbon monoxide uptake: Application of Goodpasture's syndrome, N. Engl J Med 295:1391–1396, 1976

41. Greening A, Hughes JMB. Use of carbon monoxide to monitor pulmonary haemorrhage. Thorax 33:540, 1978

8

Arterial Blood Gases: Hypoxemia and Acid-Base Balance

I. Barry Sorkin
Roberta M. Goldring

PULMONARY FUNCTION TESTS: A   ISBN 0-8089-1764-4   Copyright © 1987 by Grune & Stratton
GUIDE FOR THE STUDENT AND HOUSE OFFICER   All rights of reproduction in any form reserved.

ARTERIAL BLOOD GAS ANALYSIS

The analysis of arterial blood is divided into two broad categories: oxygenation and acid-base balance. This chapter will address evaluation of mechanisms of oxygen exchange in the normal and abnormal individual, principles by which one can distinguish pulmonary from non-pulmonary mechanisms for gas exchange abnormalities, and the identification and quantification of metabolic and respiratory acid-base disorders.

Arterial blood gas analysis involves direct measurement of three specific parameters: pH, PO_2 and PCO_2. From the pH and PO_2 one derives, through a calculation based on the oxyhemoglobin dissociation curve, the oxygen saturation. From the pH and PCO_2, through the use of the Henderson-Hasselbalch equation, one can derive the plasma bicarbonate concentration; through the use of Siggaard-Andersen nomograms, one can derive standard bicarbonate and base excess.

Sampling Arterial Blood

The three conventional sites for drawing arterial blood are the radial, brachial, and femoral arteries. The radial artery is preferred if it can be demonstrated that ulnar circulation is adequate. A simple test for this involves manual occlusion of both radial and ulnar arteries until the hand whitens. Upon release of pressure on the ulnar artery, a brisk reddening of the palm will demonstrate the presence of adequate collateral circulation.

Once the sample is withdrawn, air bubbles are expelled and the syringe is capped so that the sample remains anaerobic. Since metabolism by the cells will change the gas values, the sample should be analyzed immediately or the syringe stored in ice. When the PO_2 is above 100 torr, the metabolism of blood cells will cause a more rapid decrease in PO_2, even on ice, and analysis must be immediate. In addition, high white cell volume, as in leukemia, will accelerate the decrease in PO_2.

A variety of machines are available for blood gas measurements; many are now automated. Quality control is essential for meaningful results; the calibration may be assessed using control solutions. The sample size required for most automated analyzers is less than 0.5 ml. The blood should be inspected for clots or air bubbles and then thoroughly mixed by vigorously rotating the syringe before insertion into the analyzer.

Nomograms

Direct readings of pH, PO_2, and PCO_2 are obtained. Automated machines will print out calculated values for oxygen saturation and plasma bicarbonate, utilizing algorithms that describe the oxyhemoglobin dissociation curve (Appendix 8-1) and the Henderson-Hasselbalch equation. Appendix 8-2 illustrates an alignment nomogram for obtaining the plasma bicarbonate concentration. Standard bicarbonate, blood base excess, and extracellular base excess can also be obtained using the relationships defined by Siggaard-Andersen.[1] Appendix 8-2 yields extracellular base excess based on a simplification of the Siggaard-Andersen nomogram.

The partial pressures and pH are equilibrated to 37°C in the machine. If the patient's body temperature differs from 37°, the measured values no longer reflect those in the patient. If the machine can not be set to correct for this temperature difference, correction factors are available. Appendix 8-3 provides a useful nomogram for correcting PCO_2 and PO_2.[2,3] These corrections become clinically relevant when body temperature is above 102°F (38.9°C) or less than 97°F (36.1°C).

Measurements of Oxygen in the Blood

Oxygen is carried in the blood in two forms: dissolved in the plasma and combined with hemoglobin. The measured PO_2 quantitates the amount of oxygen dissolved in the plasma. This represents a very small amount of the total oxygen carried by the blood, since the major carrying capacity of oxygen is in the red cells. The volume of oxygen carried in 100 ml of plasma is equal to 0.003 ml for each 1 mmHg partial pressure of oxygen. Thus, the value of oxygen dissolved in plasma at a normal PO_2 of 90 torr equals 90 times 0.003 or 0.27 ml of oxygen per 100 ml of blood. Each gram of fully saturated hemoglobin carries 1.34 ml of oxygen per 100 ml of blood. Therefore, at a normal oxygen saturation of 97 percent and a hemoglobin concentration of 15 g percent, the volume of oxygen bound to hemoglobin would be equal to 1.34 times 15 times 0.97 or 19.5 ml of oxygen per 100 ml of whole blood (ml percent).

Although the PO_2 is measured in clinical practice, the extrapolation to total oxygen content provides the measure of total oxygen available for delivery to the tissues. The standard oxyhemoglobin dissociation curve is used for this purpose (Appendix 8-1). Direct measurement (rather than extrapolation) of oxygen content or saturation is desirable under certain conditions: in evaluation of shifts of the oxyhemoglobin dissociation curve and for greater accuracy when the PO_2 is below 60 torr, as in the assessment of mixed venous oxygen content.

Oxygen content and capacity may be obtained directly using the Van-Slyke apparatus, and saturation (oxyhemoglobin) is derived from these measurements. This technique requires highly skilled personnel and is not widely used currently. Oxygen saturation is usually measured directly with an oximeter. The principle of oximetry involves the measurement of selected spectral absorbance values that correspond to oxyhemoglobin, reduced hemoglobin, carboxyhemoglobin, and methemoglobin. Most oximeters yield values for oxygen saturation based on total hemoglobin that includes values for methemoglobin and carboxyhemoglobin concentration. Therefore, the *measured* oxygen saturation obtained from an oximeter differs from oxyhemoglobin saturation in the presence of significant values for methemoglobin or carboxyhemoglobin:

Equation 8-1

$$\text{oxyhemoglobin saturation} = \frac{\text{measured oxygen saturation}}{100 - (\text{COHgb} + \text{MetHgb})} \times 100$$

The *measured* oxygen saturation is used for calculation of oxygen content; oxyhemoglobin saturation is used in evaluating abnormalities of the oxyhemoglobin dissociation curve.

Oxyhemoglobin Dissociation Curve

Since oxygen delivery is a function of arterial oxygen content, the extrapolation of oxygen delivery from measured PO_2 requires the assumption that the oxyhemoglobin dissociation curve is normal in the patient to be assessed. Temperature, pH, and PCO_2 are measured and incorporated into the usual estimate of oxyhemoglobin saturation from the normal O_2 dissociation curve. In usual clinical circumstances, it is assumed that the patient has normal intracellular 2,3-DPG, phosphate, and carboxyhemoglobin concentrations and no hemoglobinopathy. If any of these factors is suspected to be abnormal, the oxyhemoglobin saturation should be measured directly, even if PaO_2 is normal, since the standard curve may not accurately predict the patient's saturation.

The P_{50} is clinically used as an assessment of the position of the oxyhemoglobin dissociation curve. It is defined as the partial pressure of the PO_2 in the plasma at 50 percent oxyhemoglobin saturation (Appendix 8-1) and can be expressed at either the pH of the patient's blood or at the standard pH of 7.4. The normal value for standard P_{50}, (at a pH of 7.4) is 26.7 ± 3 torr.

In order to obtain the P_{50}, a blood sample with a measured oxyhemoglobin saturation between 20 and 80 percent is required. If the saturation of a sample is not in this range, it may be tonometered with known gas mixtures to adjust the saturation accordingly. The PO_2, pH, and PCO_2 are measured in the usual manner, and oxygen saturation is independently measured. In the presence of methemoglobin or carboxyhemoglobin this *measured* saturation is corrected to *true* oxyhemoglobin saturation with Equation 8-1. The observed PO_2 is adjusted to standard conditions and compared to the PO_2 predicted by a normal oxyhemoglobin dissociation curve. For these calculations the following formula is used[3]:

Equation 8-2

$$P_{50} \text{ (Standard)} = \frac{26.7 \times PO_2 \text{ (Observed)}}{PO_2 \text{ (Standard)}}$$

where PO_2(observed) is the measured PO_2 adjusted to pH 7.40 and PCO_2 40 at 37°C; PO_2(standard) is the PO_2 predicted from the measured oxyhemoglobin saturation at pH 7.40 and PCO_2 40; 26.7 is the normal P_{50} at pH 7.40. Equations for PO_2(observed) and PO_2(standard) are described in references 8 and 3.

EVALUATION OF ARTERIAL OXYGENATION

Introduction

Identification of the underlying mechanisms causing impaired oxygenation is key to proper diagnosis and management. The abnormality must be quantified, and changing clinical conditions (in the FIO_2 or in the patient's hemoglobin and cardiac output) should be reflected. Finally, clinical measures of oxygenation must be readily accessible if they are to be used at the bedside. The goal of this section is to provide a framework for use of the following parameters: arterial PO_2, oxygen saturation, alveolar-arterial PO_2 gradient and calculated shunt.

Arterial PO$_2$ (PaO$_2$)

The PaO$_2$ reflects the overall effectiveness of the lungs in oxygenating blood. Arterial blood comprises a mixture of pulmonary end-capillary blood draining the many alveolar units. Thus, the simple measure of oxygenation, PaO$_2$, is actually the result of the complex manner in which blood from various regions of the lung mixes to form the arterial blood.

There are major limitations in the use of PaO$_2$ to quantify an oxygenation defect. These limitations are the result of the fact that the PaO$_2$ actually represents a small portion of the total oxygen transported by the blood; most of the oxygen is combined with hemoglobin. Also, since the oxyhemoglobin dissociation curve is curvilinear, any change in PaO$_2$ has a very different meaning at different points along the curve. For example, the improvement from a PaO$_2$ of 40 to 60 torr represents a more significant quantitative change in oxygenation than one from 60 to 80 torr. The concepts of alveolar-arterial PO$_2$ gradient and calculated total and "anatomic" shunt were developed[4] to identify and better quantify the oxygenation defect. Alveolar-arterial PO$_2$ gradient is useful to identify the presence of an intra-pulmonary defect in oxygenation. Calculated shunt provides a more quantitative measure since it incorporates hemoglobin concentration, pH, arterial and mixed venous oxygen content, and cardiac output. The next sections will define these parameters and present a practical approach to their application.

Ideal Alveolar PO$_2$ (Ideal PAO$_2$)

The oxygen content of pulmonary capillary blood is determined by the oxygen tension of the alveolar air with which it communicates. Thus, PaO$_2$ must be related to PAO$_2$ in order to evaluate the oxygenation function of the lung. Regional variations in matching of ventilation to perfusion exist, even in the normal lung, resulting in nonuniformity of PAO$_2$ and, therefore, end-capillary PO$_2$. The PaO$_2$ is derived from the mixture of blood draining these end-capillaries. The calculation of ideal PAO$_2$ provides a reference for evaluation of PaO$_2$. The ideal PAO$_2$ is the oxygen tension that would exist in all gas exchanging alveoli if ventilation/perfusion relationships were totally uniform and if the PCO$_2$ were equal to measured arterial.

Figure 8-1 illustrates the use of this concept in the evaluation of arterial oxygenation. The diagram includes two compartments. One compartment is ideal end-capillary blood in equilibrium with ideal alveolar gas. If all of the mixed venous blood flowed through this compartment, then PaO$_2$ would equal ideal alveolar. Even in the normal individual, however, the PaO$_2$ is lower than the ideal PAO$_2$. The other compartment in the figure represents the mixed venous blood flow that would have to mix with the ideal end-capillary blood to produce the measured PaO$_2$ in a given patient. The mechanisms that contribute to this venous-like admixture during room air breathing include ventilation/perfusion imbalance, diffusion limitation, and "anatomic" shunt as illustrated.

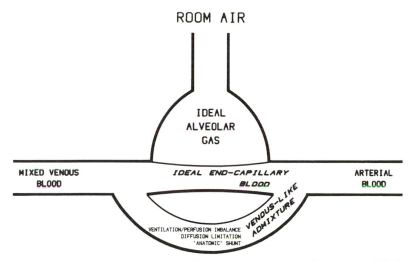

Fig. 8-1. Schematic illustrating venous-like admixture based on the concept of ideal alveolar gas during room air breathing.

The venous-like admixture results in a defect in oxygenation that is identified by relating measured arterial blood gas composition to calculated ideal alveolar gas composition. The defect can be expressed in two different ways: A-a PO_2 gradient (utilizing oxygen tension) or calculated shunt (as a function of oxygen content). Both measures require the calculation of ideal alveolar PO_2.

The ideal PAO_2 is calculated by use of the alveolar air equation:

Equation 8-3a

$$PAO_2 = PIO_2 - \frac{PACO_2}{R}$$

This calculation requires the inspired PO_2 (PIO_2), and a measured or assumed respiratory exchange ratio (R). In accord with the definition of ideal alveolar gas, $PACO_2$ is assumed equal to $PaCO_2$. Thus PAO_2 is lower than the PIO_2 because of the presence of alveolar PCO_2. The use of R corrects the PCO_2 for the effect of the small difference in volume between inspired and expired gas. If R is not measured directly, a value of 0.8 is generally assumed when the patient is breathing room air, and a value of 1 when breathing at an FIO_2 of 1.00. The PIO_2 reflects the partial pressure of oxygen of humidified, inspired gas before it reaches gas-exchanging alveoli. This number is calculated from the inspired fraction of oxygen (FIO_2) and dry barometric pressure as follows:

Equation 8-3b

$$PIO_2 = FIO_2 \times (\text{Barometric pressure} - 47)$$

On breathing room air at standard barometric pressure the PIO_2 equals approximately 149 torr. Substituting into the alveolar air equation (Equation 8-3a) 149 torr for the PIO_2, 40 torr for the $PaCO_2$, and 0.8 for R, the normal ideal PAO_2 during room air breathing equals approximately 100 torr.

The form of the alveolar air equation presented (Equation 8-3a) is adequate for most clinical purposes; however, it actually represents a simplification of a more accurate equation which has been used in the preparation of data for the figures and tables of this chapter:

Equation 8-3c

$$PAO_2 = PIO_2 - PaCO_2\left(FIO_2 + \frac{(1 - FIO_2)}{R}\right)$$

Alveolar–Arterial PO_2 Gradient (A-a PO_2)

The A-a PO_2 gradient is the PO_2 difference between the calculated ideal alveolar gas (Equation 8-3a) and the measured arterial blood:

Equation 8-3d

$$\text{A-a } PO_2 = \text{Alveolar } PO_2 - \text{Arterial } PO_2$$

This gradient identifies the presence of *venous-like admixture* and, therefore, of an intrapulmonary or intracardiac defect in oxygenation. The underlying mechanisms that may contribute to this venous-like admixture include ventilation/perfusion imbalance, diffusion limitation, and "anatomic" shunt (Fig. 8-1). A measurable A-a PO_2 gradient exists even in the normal subject. On room air breathing the normal range is about 10 to 20 torr in the young adult (up to 30 torr in subjects over 60 years of age).

An abnormally increased A-a PO_2 marks the presence of an intrinsic pulmonary abnormality and is, therefore, an important clinical tool. However, because PO_2 does not relate to oxygen content in a linear manner (as defined by the oxyhemoglobin dissociation curve), a given A-a PO_2 gradient at a constant FIO_2 reflects a different magnitude of abnormality at different PaO_2 levels. The use of the calculated shunt provides an important advantage since it is based upon oxygen content and, therefore, quantitates the abnormality.

Calculated Shunt

Definitions

The calculated shunt quantitates venous-like admixture. Calculated shunt is defined as the percentage of the cardiac output that would have to contribute to ideal end-capillary blood as venous-like admixture in order to account for the observed arterial oxygen saturation at a given FIO_2. An estimated oxygen content of ideal

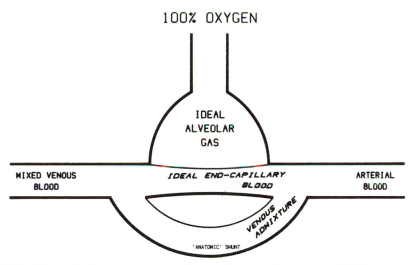

Fig. 8-2. Schematic illustrating venous admixture based on the concept of ideal alveolar gas during 100 percent oxygen breathing.

end-capillary blood as well as the measured oxygen content of arterial and mixed venous blood are required. In this manner, calculated shunt integrates hemoglobin concentration and cardiac output and allows for a quantitative estimate of venous-like admixture during room air breathing or at any level of FIO_2.

Total shunt. When room air is inspired, the venous-like admixture is calculated as though it were a true shunt and is referred to as *total shunt.* This quantitates the same mechanisms that determine the A-a PO_2 gradient: ventilation/perfusion imbalance, diffusion limitation, and "anatomic" shunt (see Fig. 8-1.).

Normal values for total shunt range from 3 to 8 percent in the young adult and may increase to 15 percent in the older population.

"Anatomic" shunt. The venous-like admixture as quantitated by the calculated shunt decreases with increasing FIO_2. The change in calculated shunt between room air and an FIO_2 of 1.00 is due to the decreased contribution of ventilation/perfusion imbalance and diffusion limitation. Figure 8-2 illustrates the residual oxygenation defect at an FIO_2 of 1.00, which defines venous admixture and is termed *"anatomic" shunt.* This may represent a *true* anatomic shunt (e.g. intracardiac or intrapulmonary right-to-left shunt) or a *virtual* "anatomic" shunt due to intrapulmonary perfusion of unventilated alveoli. The normal range for "anatomic" shunt is 2 to 4 percent of the cardiac output.

Confusion arises because of variations in shunt nomenclature. On room air breathing, total shunt is a commonly used term to describe the calculated shunt; other terms are often used: physiologic shunt, functional shunt, and venous-like admixture. When the FIO_2 is 1.00, terms that frequently substitute for "anatomic" shunt include venous admixture, residual shunt, virtual shunt, frank shunt, right-to-left shunt and, even, just plain shunt. On intermediate levels of FIO_2, the least confusing term is, simply, calculated shunt.

The Shunt Equation

The shunt equation is a mixing equation based on the assumption that the total amount of oxygen transported in the arterial blood is equal to the sum of oxygen flowing through the ideal end-capillary and the shunt compartments. If $\dot{Q}_T$ represents cardiac output, $\dot{Q}_S$ represents shunt blood flow, and $(\dot{Q}_T - \dot{Q}_S)$ represents ideal end-capillary blood flow, then oxygen transport is expressed as follows:

Equation 8-4a

$\dot{Q}_T \times$ Arterial O_2 content $=$

$[(\dot{Q}_T - \dot{Q}_S) \times$ Ideal end-capillary O_2 content$] + [\dot{Q}_S \times$ Mixed venous O_2 content$]$

A rearrangement yields the standard shunt formula:

Equation 8-4b

$$\frac{\dot{Q}_S}{\dot{Q}_T} = \frac{\text{Ideal end-capillary } O_2 \text{ content} - \text{Arterial } O_2 \text{ content}}{\text{Ideal end-capillary } O_2 \text{ content} - \text{Mixed venous } O_2 \text{ content}}$$

The numerator of the shunt equation is the difference in oxygen content between ideally oxygenated end-capillary blood and the observed arterial blood; this decrease in oxygen content reflects the effect of venous-like admixture. The denominator is the difference in oxygen content between ideally oxygenated end-capillary blood and mixed venous blood; this reflects the increase in oxygen content that would occur in transit across the lung in the absence of any venous-like admixture. The ratio of these oxygen content changes is equivalent to the fraction of the cardiac output that would have to contribute as venous-like admixture to the ideal end-capillary blood flow to account for the observed arterial oxygen content.

The above calculation of shunt, at any level FIO_2, requires estimates of arterial, mixed venous and ideal end-capillary oxygen content. The oxygen content in each compartment is equal to the oxygen bound to the hemoglobin plus the oxygen dissolved in the plasma. The bound oxygen content is equal to the oxygen saturation times the oxygen combining power of hemoglobin (Hgb $\times$ 1.34). The dissolved oxygen equals the PO_2 times the solubility coefficient of oxygen in plasma (0.003). The equations for arterial, mixed venous, and ideal end-capillary oxygen content (in ml percent) are listed below in Equation 8-5.

Equation 8-5

Arterial O_2 content (ml%) $=$

(Arterial Sat/100 $\times$ 1.34 $\times$ Hgb) $+$ (Arterial PO_2 $\times$ 0.003)

Mixed venous O_2 content (ml%) $=$

(Mixed venous Sat/100 $\times$ 1.34 $\times$ Hgb) $+$ (Mixed venous PO_2 $\times$ 0.003)

Ideal end-capillary O_2 content (ml%) =

(Ideal end-capillary Sat/100 × 1.34 × Hgb) + (Alveolar PAO_2 × 0.003)

Since mixed venous (pulmonary arterial) blood is not always available, normal values for (a-v̄) O_2 content difference of 4–5 vol percent may be assumed if clinically appropriate.

To calculate the ideal end-capillary oxygen content, the end-capillary PO_2 is assumed equal to the ideal PAO_2, which is calculated in the standard manner (Equation 8-3a). This number is then converted to oxygen saturation using arterial pH and the standard oxyhemoglobin dissociation curve (Appendix 8-1 or Reference 7). If the calculated PAO_2 is greater than 150 torr, ideal end-capillary saturation can be assumed to be 100 percent.

Simplified Shunt Equation

An alternative to the above calculations is a simplified version of the shunt equation (Equation 8-6) that is valid when the ideal PAO_2 is greater than 150 torr.[5] This condition is usually satisfied when the FIO_2 is greater than 0.35.

Equation 8-6

$$\frac{\dot{Q}_S}{\dot{Q}_T} = \frac{(PAO_2 - PaO_2) \times 0.003}{(a-\bar{v})\ O_2\ \text{content difference} + (PAO_2 - PaO_2) \times 0.003}$$

Shunt Nomograms

Nomograms are available to estimate the calculated shunt (see Appendices 8-4 and 8-5), based on the standard shunt equation (Equation 8-4b).

Appendix 8-4 is a simple nomogram that assumes standard conditions: pH 7.40, hemoglobin 12 gm percent, and arterio-venous O_2 content difference 5 ml percent (cardiac output normal). Variations in pH and hemoglobin concentration affect its accuracy.

Appendix 8-5 is a more complex nomogram for calculation of shunt in the patient whose cardiac output is abnormal and provides for alterations in hemoglobin.

The Arterial/Alveolar (a/A) PO_2 Ratio

The ratio of the PaO_2 to the ideal PAO_2 is a measure of oxygenation that is sometimes used as an alternative to calculation of A-a gradient or shunt. Its usefulness stems from its simplicity and from the fact that it remains relatively constant with variations in FIO_2. This allows for comparison of blood gases at different FIO_2 as well as prediction of the PaO_2 at a new FIO_2. Normally, the a/A PO_2 ratio is greater than 0.75. The conditions under which this ratio actually remains constant are limited and impose constraints on its clinical use: the FIO_2 must be greater than 0.35, and the PaO_2 must be less than 100 torr.[6]

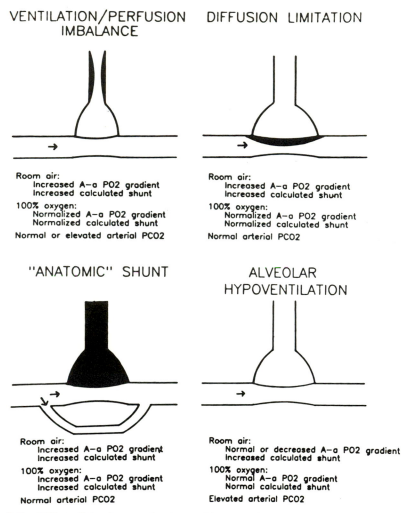

VENTILATION/PERFUSION IMBALANCE

Room air:
   Increased A—a PO2 gradient
   Increased calculated shunt
100% oxygen:
   Normalized A—a PO2 gradient
   Normalized calculated shunt
Normal or elevated arterial PCO2

DIFFUSION LIMITATION

Room air:
   Increased A—a PO2 gradient
   Increased calculated shunt
100% oxygen:
   Normalized A—a PO2 gradient
   Normalized calculated shunt
Normal arterial PCO2

"ANATOMIC" SHUNT

Room air:
   Increased A—a PO2 gradient
   Increased calculated shunt
100% oxygen:
   Increased A—a PO2 gradient
   Increased calculated shunt
Normal arterial PCO2

ALVEOLAR HYPOVENTILATION

Room air:
   Normal or decreased A—a PO2 gradient
   Increased calculated shunt
100% oxygen:
   Normal A—a PO2 gradient
   Normal calculated shunt
Elevated arterial PCO2

Fig. 8-3. Effect of the four mechanisms of hypoxemia on A-a PO_2 gradient, calculated shunt and $PaCO_2$.

MECHANISMS OF HYPOXEMIA

Definitions

This section describes the four major mechanisms responsible for arterial hypoxemia. These mechanisms are depicted in Figure 8-3 and include ventilation/perfusion imbalance, diffusion limitation, "anatomic" shunt, and alveolar hypoventilation. All result in reductions of PaO_2 and oxygen saturation. Ventilation/perfusion imbalance, diffusion limitation, and "anatomic" shunt reflect hypoxemia caused by intrinsic pulmonary abnormalities. Alveolar hypoventilation, however, need not reflect an abnormal intrapulmonary mechanism but may be the result of a change in overall ventilation with normal lung function.

Ventilation/Perfusion Imbalance

This mechanism for arterial hypoxemia results from variations in matching of ventilation to perfusion. In alveolar units where ventilation is low relative to perfusion, the PO_2 will be reduced relative to the ideal PAO_2. The pulmonary end-capillary blood that is in equilibrium with the reduced PAO_2 in these units contributes as venous-like admixture (see Fig. 8-1), which results in arterial hypoxemia. When the FIO_2 is 1.00, the variations in alveolar and end-capillary PO_2 that are present during room air breathing are minimized as a result of nitrogen washout. Venous-like admixture and the resultant arterial hypoxemia due to all mechanisms except "anatomic" shunt are eliminated at FIO_2 1.00 because of uniformly high levels of PAO_2. Thus A-a PO_2 gradient and calculated shunt will be increased on room air breathing and normalized at FIO_2 1.00.

Diffusion Limitation

This abnormality is defined by arterial hypoxemia that results (during room air breathing) from the incomplete equilibration of alveolar gas with pulmonary end-capillary blood. This incomplete equilibration can be the result of a thickened alveolar-capillary membrane or a decreased pulmonary capillary transit time. Transit time may, in turn, be reduced due to a smaller pulmonary vascular bed, at rest, or as a result of increased cardiac output, as during exercise. When the FIO_2 is 1.00, the reduced PO_2 in the end-capillaries rises to levels that effectively saturate end-capillary blood because the greatly increased PAO_2 overcomes diffusion limitation. Thus, the venous-like admixture and the resultant hypoxemia from diffusion limitation are eliminated with high FIO_2 by the increased driving pressure for oxygen.

Although ventilation/perfusion ($\dot{V}/\dot{Q}$) balance and diffusion limitation are defined as distinct and separate causes for hypoxemia, blood gas analysis cannot distinguish one from the other. $\dot{V}/\dot{Q}$ imbalance is an important cause of hypoxemia in pulmonary disease. It is controversial whether hypoxemia results from diffusion limitation under resting conditions, even in disease. However, during exercise, diffusion limitation may become clinically important. Since diffusion limitation cannot be distinguished from $\dot{V}/\dot{Q}$ imbalance by using the A-a PO_2 gradient or calculated shunt, any contribution of diffusion limitation is incorporated into the quantitation of the abnormality by these methods of analysis. Moreover, measurements of diffusing capacity (D_LCO) may not separate these mechanisms since this test is influenced by $\dot{V}/\dot{Q}$ imbalance (See Chapter 9). Conversely, a low D_LCO may not be associated with abnormal resting PaO_2.

"Anatomic" Shunt

"Anatomic" shunt represents the venous admixture resulting from mixed venous blood flow through unventilated areas. It is identified as the residual defect in oxygenation at FIO_2 1.00 (See Fig. 8-2). In the normal, "anatomic" shunt represents the percentage of the cardiac output flowing through veno-arterial communications within the heart and lungs. Most of this shunt is accounted for by the drainage from the Thebesian veins into the left atrium and by pulmonary blood flowing directly from bronchial to pulmonary veins. The normal value for this "anatomic" shunt rarely exceeds 2 to 4 percent of the cardiac output. However, disease processes that are associated with collapse or non-ventilation of perfused alveoli are characterized by an oxygenation defect that is not obliterated with FIO_2 1.00. This abnormal "anatomic" shunt is quantitated by the value of the calculated shunt at FIO_2 1.00.

Identification of "anatomic" shunt requires washout of nitrogen from the lungs. This is complete in the normal subject after about 5 minutes at FIO_2 1.00. In a patient with obstructive airway disease, nitrogen washout may require as long as 20 minutes.

Alveolar Hypoventilation

An elevated $PaCO_2$ is the hallmark of alveolar hypoventilation. This abnormality is defined by an increase in $PACO_2$ that results in a decreased PAO_2. This change in alveolar gas composition may be a result of an extrapulmonary reduction in total ventilation, or an intrapulmonary abnormality in ventilation/perfusion imbalance. The latter may occur despite high levels of total ventilation when intrinsic disease leads to large areas where ventilation exceeds perfusion leading to increased dead space ventilation (see *Mechanisms of Hypercapnia* below). Both mechanisms are identified by an increased $PaCO_2$.

Arterial hypoxemia is the obligatory result of alveolar hypoventilation since increase in $PACO_2$ results in reduction of PAO_2. This inverse relationship between PAO_2 and $PACO_2$ is expressed in the alveolar air equation (Equation 8-3a). Therefore, if the PCO_2 is elevated, one of the mechanisms responsible for hypoxemia is alveolar hypoventilation. However, associated or coincidental lung disease can also contribute to the oxygenation abnormality through one of the other mechanisms. To evaluate whether hypoventilation is the sole mechanism for the hypoxemia, the A-a PO_2 gradient and calculated shunt become important tools. These measures of oxygenation should remain within normal limits in the absence of lung disease and should become elevated in presence of intrinsic pulmonary abnormality.

In the absence of intrinsic pulmonary disease, the assumption that both A-a PO_2 gradient and shunt remain unchanged as $PaCO_2$ rises, must be qualified. When "pure" alveolar hypoventilation is present during room air breathing, the A-a PO_2 gradient will, in fact, be normal or slightly decreased. If hypoventilation is severe, the calculated shunt will become elevated: values for calculated shunt may approach 15–20 percent as $PaCO_2$ values approach 80 torr. Therefore, when alveolar hypoventilation is present, guidelines for using shunt to identify an associated gas exchange abnormality are difficult to define precisely. It has not been clearly established whether this increase in calculated shunt is a reflection of a diffusion limitation imposed by lowered PAO_2. However, an elevated total shunt that is associated with an elevated A-a PO_2 gradient remains a reliable marker of intrinsic disease despite the level of $PaCO_2$.

In the presence of alveolar hyperventilation, when $PACO_2$ is low, there is a corresponding increase in PAO_2. This results in an increased PaO_2. Thus, a "normal" PaO_2, when $PaCO_2$ is reduced may, in fact, mask an intrinsic oxygenation abnormality. Identification of an increased A-a PO_2 gradient in this setting confirms the presence of an abnormality.

Effect of Increasing Inspired Oxygen in the Normal Subject

Figure 8-4 illustrates the changes in PaO_2, A-a PO_2 gradient, and calculated shunt over the full range of FIO_2 from room air to 1.00 under normal conditions. During room air breathing, the PaO_2 of 90 torr is typical of young, healthy adults. The A-a gradient of 12 torr reflects a normal total shunt of 4 percent. At the other end of the scale, the PaO_2 at FIO_2 1.00 has increased linearly to 623 torr. This demonstrates the ease with which increases in FIO_2 raise the PaO_2 in the normal lung.

Associated with the linear increase in PaO_2 between FIO_2 0.21 and 1.00, the A-a PO_2 gradient has *increased* to 50 torr at an FIO_2 of about 0.50 and then remains essentially constant between an FIO_2 of 0.50 and 1.00. In contrast, calculated shunt *decreases* between FIO_2 0.21 and 0.50 and remains essentially constant between 0.50 and 1.00. This apparent contradiction is the result of the nonlinearity of the oxyhemoglobin dissociation curve.

The nonlinearity of the oxyhemoglobin dissociation curve dictates that the interrelationships between A-a PO_2 gradient and shunt vary depending on the level of FIO_2. When PO_2 values are below 100 torr, the oxyhemoglobin dissociation curve is steep; at PO_2 values above 100 torr, the curve is relatively flat. The FIO_2 determines the PAO_2, and the venous-like admixture determines the PaO_2; the difference between ideal alveolar and arterial oxygen tension (A-a PO_2 gradient) depends on the steepness of oxyhemoglobin dissociation curve where these points fall. Figures 8-5 and 8-6 are used to illustrate this phenomenon. Figure 8-5 illus-

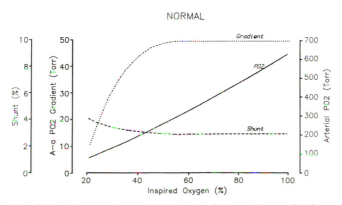

Fig. 8-4. Changes in arterial PO_2, A-a PO_2 gradient and calculated shunt with increasing inspired oxygen in the normal individual.

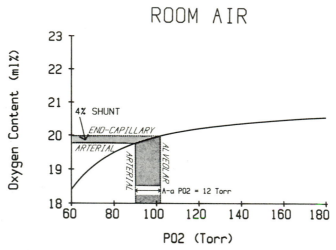

Fig. 8-5. Segment of oxyhemoglobin dissociation curve (Hgb = 15 Gm percent) illustrating effect of normal venous-like admixture on A-a PO_2 gradient while breathing room air. Total shunt of 4 percent results in A-a PO_2 of 12 torr on the relatively steep segment of the curve.

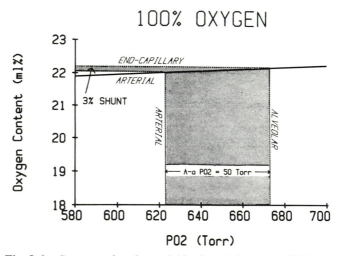

Fig. 8-6. Segment of oxyhemoglobin dissociation curve (Hgb = 15 Gm percent) illustrating effect of normal venous admixture on A-a PO_2 gradient while breathing 100 percent oxygen. "Anatomic" shunt of 3 percent results in A-a PO_2 of 50 torr on the relatively flat segment of the curve.

trates the effect of the normal 4 percent total shunt on the A-a PO_2 gradient during room air breathing when the PO_2 values fall on the steep portion of the oxyhemoglobin dissociation curve. The ideal end-capillary O_2 content is 20 ml percent at the ideal PAO_2 of 102 torr. The arterial oxygen content is 19.7 ml percent at a PO_2 of 90 torr and is a result of the venous-like admixture to the ideal end-capillary blood flow. This oxygen content change from ideal end-capillary to arterial results in the normal A-a PO_2 gradient of 12 torr.

Figure 8-6 illustrates the effect of the normal 3 percent "anatomic" shunt on the A-a PO_2 gradient at FIO_2 1.00 when the PO_2 values fall on the flat portion of oxyhemoglobin dissociation curve. The ideal end-capillary O_2 content is now 22.2 ml percent at the ideal PAO_2 of 673 torr (due largely to the increase in dissolved oxygen). The arterial oxygen content is 22.2 ml percent at a PO_2 of 623 and is the result of the venous admixture to ideal end-capillary blood flow. This oxygen content change from ideal end-capillary to arterial results in the normal A-a PO_2 gradient of 50 torr at FIO_2 1.00. This is larger than the A-a PO_2 gradient during room air breathing (caused by a similar magnitude of shunt) because of the change in shape of the dissociation curve.

To evaluate the clinical significance of a calculated A-a PO_2 gradient it is necessary to compare the A-a PO_2 gradient to the predicted normal gradient at the *same* FIO_2 and to evaluate venous-like admixture by calculating shunt.

Evaluation of Oxygenation in Disease

A systematic approach to quantifying the abnormalities in oxygenation and to understanding the mechanisms responsible for them will be presented. Clinical examples will be used to illustrate the four major mechanisms. Each example will include the range of values for PaO_2, A-a PO_2 gradient and calculated shunt for inspired oxygen levels from room air to FIO_2 1.00. The PaO_2 on room air in each example is 50 torr. This is to emphasize the fact that entirely different underlying abnormalities may be responsible for the same PaO_2.

Ventilation/Perfusion Imbalance and Diffusion Limitation

The identification of ventilation/perfusion imbalance and/or diffusion limitation requires that any defect in oxygenation will be obliterated at an FIO_2 of 1.00.

Figure 8-7 illustrates the changes in PaO_2, A-a PO_2 gradient and calculated shunt that correspond to increases in FIO_2 in a patient with a PaO_2 of 50 torr during room air breathing due to ventilation/perfusion imbalance and/or diffusion abnormality. The $PaCO_2$ is assumed normal at 40 torr. At the room air level the A-a PO_2 gradient is calculated (from Equation 8-3d) to be 52 torr; the total shunt of 36 percent is calculated (Equation 8-4b) or read from a nomogram (Appendix 8-4 or 8-5) based on a normal (a-$\bar{v}$) O_2 content difference of 5 vol percent.

With increasing FIO_2 between 0.21 and 0.50, there is a relatively small change in PaO_2; above FIO_2 0.50, the PaO_2 increases in normal fashion to 623 torr at FIO_2 1.00. The calculated A-a PO_2 gradient increases between FIO_2 0.21 and 0.50 and

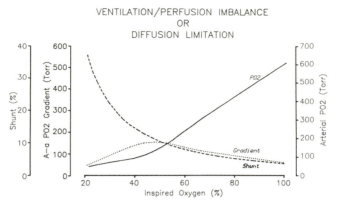

Fig. 8-7. Changes in arterial PO_2, A-a PO_2 gradient and calculated shunt with increasing inspired oxygen when abnormality of ventilation/perfusion or diffusion is the mechanism of hypoxemia. Arterial $PO_2 = 50$ torr on room air breathing.

then decreases to a normal value at $FIO_2 = 1.00$. Despite the initial increase in the A-a PO_2 gradient, the calculated shunt decreases; the major decrease in shunt occurs between FIO_2 0.21 and 0.50, in this example, with a small further decrease between FIO_2 0.50 and 1.00. The unique distribution of $\dot{V}/\dot{Q}$ inequalities within the lungs of a given patient dictates the manner in which venous-like admixture (as quantitated by calculated shunt) decreases with FIO_2.

This example summarizes the principles used in confirming $\dot{V}/\dot{Q}$ imbalance or diffusion limitation as the predominant mechanism for hypoxemia. On room air the A-a PO_2 gradient is widened and reflects an elevated total shunt. With increasing FIO_2 this abnormality is obliterated and is reflected in a normal "anatomic" shunt at FIO_2 1.00.

"Anatomic" Shunt

The demonstration of "anatomic" shunt requires a persistent oxygenation abnormality at an FIO_2 of 1.00.

Figure 8-8 illustrates the changes in PaO_2, A-a PO_2 gradient, and calculated shunt that correspond to increases in FIO_2 in a patient with "anatomic" shunt as the primary abnormality. During room air breathing the PaO_2 is (as in the previous example) 50 torr. $PaCO_2$ is assumed normal at 40 torr. The A-a PO_2 gradient is 52 torr and reflects a total shunt (read from Appendix 8-4) of 36 percent at an arteriovenous O_2 content difference of 5 vol percent. At the upper end of the scale, the PaO_2 at FIO_2 1.00 has increased to only 90 torr. The A-a PO_2 gradient continues to increase with increasing FIO_2 to a level of 583 torr. This widened A-a PO_2 gradient at FIO_2 1.00 marks the presence of "anatomic" shunt. The calculated value of 33 percent is similar to the total shunt of 36 percent on room air breathing.

If "anatomic" shunt is the sole mechanism for hypoxemia on room air, then the calculated shunt at any level of FIO_2 between room air and 1.00 will remain almost

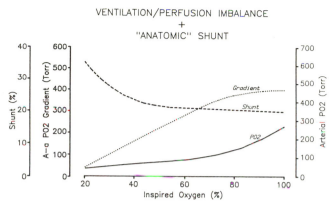

Fig. 8-8. Changes in arterial PO₂, A-a PO₂ gradient and calculated shunt with increasing inspired oxygen when abnormality of "anatomic" shunt is the mechanism of hypoxemia. Arterial PO₂ = 50 torr on room air breathing.

constant (as illustrated in Figure 8-8). Moreover, when "anatomic" shunt is greater than 40 percent, almost no change in PaO_2 should be expected for relatively large changes in FIO_2. Thus, a patient with a very reduced PaO_2 at an FIO_2 of 1.00 often tolerates large reductions in FIO_2 without a significant reduction in PaO_2.

Combined Disorder: Ventilation/Perfusion Imbalance and "Anatomic" Shunt

As in the previous examples, the PaO_2 on room air is 50 torr, and the $PaCO_2$ is assumed normal at 40 torr. (Fig. 8-9). The A-a PO₂ gradient on room air is widened at 52 torr and represents the same abnormal total shunt of 36 percent. At FIO_2 1.00,

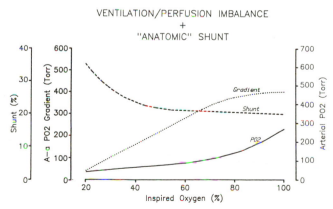

Fig. 8-9. Changes in arterial PO₂, A-a PO₂ gradient and calculated shunt when a combined abnormality of ventilation/perfusion imbalance and "anatomic" shunt is the mechanism for hypoxemia. Arterial PO₂ = 50 torr on room air breathing.

the PaO_2 has increased only to 277 torr. The A-a gradient remains widened at 396 torr and represents an "anatomic" shunt of 20 percent. The reduction in calculated shunt from 36 percent on room air to 20 percent at FIO_2 1.00 indicates that ventilation/perfusion imbalance has also contributed to the hypoxemia on room air. If "anatomic" shunt were the sole cause, there would be no reduction in calculated shunt with increase in FIO_2. It follows that the greater the decrease in calculated shunt with increasing FIO_2, the greater the contribution of ventilation/perfusion imbalance to hypoxemia.

An examination of the shunt profile indicates that even in this complex disorder, by the time FIO_2 is increased to 0.60, the calculated shunt has stabilized to a level approximating the "anatomic" shunt. Since this is the rule in most disorders, one can predict PaO_2 at a new FIO_2 (in the range between 0.60–1.00) by assuming a constant calculated shunt. One should not assume constant values for shunt at an FIO_2 below 0.50–0.60 where the added contribution from ventilation/perfusion imbalance may cause calculated shunt to increase and the predicted PO_2 to be overestimated.

Alveolar Hypoventilation

Alveolar hypoventilation results in alveolar hypoxia and, thus, provides a mechanism for arterial hypoxemia whether or not there is associated lung disease.

Table 8-1 lists blood gases on room air and at FIO_2 1.00 illustrating alveolar hypoventilation in a patient without intrinsic lung disease and with a reduced total minute ventilation. In this example, the $PaCO_2$ is acutely elevated to 78 torr. On room air the result of this degree of hypercapnia is to lower the ideal PAO_2 to 56 torr. This results in the same PaO_2 of 50 torr used in the previous examples. The A-a PO_2 gradient of 6 torr is within normal limits. The total shunt of 20 percent is elevated when compared to the normal range of 3–8 percent. However, since the elevation of shunt is associated with a normal A-a PO_2 gradient it does not reflect underlying disease but is secondary to the severe alveolar hypoventilation. In addition, at FIO_2 1.00, the PaO_2 has increased to 586 torr. The A-a gradient of 50 now represents a normal "anatomic" shunt of 3 percent.

When an increased calculated shunt is present on room air in a patient with severe alveolar hypoventilation, the distinction between a purely functional defect secondary to the hypoventilation (see earlier section, *Alveolar Hypoventilation*) versus an intrinsic pulmonary abnormality may be difficult. However, a normal or

Table 8-1
Alveolar Hypoventilation

Inspired O_2 (%)	Alveolar PO_2 (torr)	Arterial PCO_2 (torr)	Arterial PO_2 (torr)	Arterial O_2 Sat (%)	A-a PO_2 Gradient (torr)	Calculated Shunt (%)
21	56	78	50	73.4	6	20
100	635	78	586	99.9	50	3

Table 8-2
Alveolar Hypoventilation Plus Ventilation/Perfusion Imbalance

Inspired O_2 (%)	Alveolar PO_2 (torr)	Arterial PCO_2 (torr)	Arterial PO_2 (torr)	Arterial O_2 Sat (%)	A-a PO_2 Gradient (torr)	Calculated Shunt (%)
21	85	55	50	80	34	38
100	658	55	574	100	84	5

decreased A-a PO_2 gradient in the presence of elevated $PaCO_2$ remains the marker of "pure" alveolar hypoventilation.

Combined Disorder: Alveolar Hypoventilation and
Ventilation/Perfusion Imbalance

Table 8-2 lists the blood gases that might be present when intrinsic pulmonary disease is associated with hypercapnia. Since the $PaCO_2$ on room air is elevated at 55 torr, hypoventilation is present. The widened A-a PO_2 gradient of 34 torr on room air marks the presence of coexisting intrinsic pulmonary abnormality which is quantified by the total shunt of 38 percent. At FIO_2 1.00, the PaO_2 shows an increase to 574 torr, and the A-a gradient of 84 torr reflects a normalized "anatomic" shunt of 5 percent. This obliteration of venous-like admixture confirms ventilation/perfusion ($\dot{V}/\dot{Q}$) imbalance as an important mechanism for the hypoxemia on room air. An elevated total shunt that is associated with a widened A-a PO_2 gradient in the hypercapneic patient marks the presence of an intrinsic pulmonary abnormality.

MECHANISMS OF HYPERCAPNIA

CO_2 Production and Elimination

The clearance of CO_2 from the body is controlled by the respiratory system. The PCO_2 of arterial blood is an index of the effectiveness of the ventilatory system in adjusting CO_2 clearance by the lungs to metabolic production. Deviation of steady state $PaCO_2$ below 36 torr represents alveolar hyperventilation relative to tissue CO_2 production; $PaCO_2$ levels above 44 torr represent alveolar hypoventilation.

Total minute ventilation is the sum of "effective" alveolar ventilation and physiologic dead space ventilation. *"Effective" alveolar ventilation* is the component of ventilation to perfused alveoli which controls the rate of CO_2 eliminated; *physiologic dead space ventilation* includes the portion of ventilation to the conducting airways (anatomic dead space) and to alveoli that are ineffective in clearing CO_2 (alveolar dead space).

The basic relationship between $PaCO_2$ and alveolar ventilation is as follows:

Equation 8-7

$$\text{Arterial PCO}_2 = \frac{\text{CO}_2 \text{ production}}{\text{Alveolar ventilation}}$$

At a constant level of CO_2 production, $PaCO_2$ is inversely related to the level of alveolar ventilation. Figure 8-10 illustrates this relationship at a normal level of CO_2 production (100 ml/min/m²). Alveolar ventilation of 2 to 2.5 l/min/m² should result in a normal $PaCO_2$ of 40 torr. The curvilinear nature of the relationship dictates that as $PaCO_2$ rises, smaller decreases in ventilation result in more rapid increases in $PaCO_2$.

It is inherent in Equation 8-7 that elevations in $PaCO_2$ may result from either increased levels of CO_2 production or from decreased levels of alveolar ventilation. Hypermetabolic states that may contribute to elevated CO_2 production include: hyperthyroidism, elevated body temperature, septic shock, hyperalimentation, and exercise. These conditions rarely result in hypercapnia in a resting patient without intrinsic lung disease. During exercise, large increases in CO_2 production occur, but in the normal individual this is matched by an appropriate increase in alveolar ventilation, and $PaCO_2$ remains close to normal. However, in the patient with lung disease or an abnormality of ventilatory control, these elevations in CO_2 production are more likely to result in hypercapnia both at rest and during exercise.

Reduction in "effective" alveolar ventilation may occur in the presence or absence of intrinsic lung disease. In the absence of intrinsic disease, reduced alveolar ventilation results from reduced total minute ventilation or from normal minute ventilation when produced by rapid, shallow breathing. Underlying disorders are

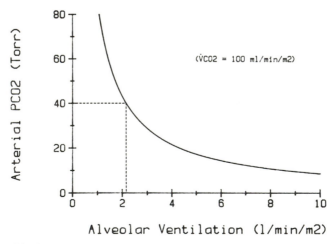

Fig. 8-10. Relationship between alveolar ventilation and $PaCO_2$. Carbon dioxide production assumed normal at 100 ml/min/m².

those of the central nervous system, neuromuscular transmission, and musculoskeletal apparatus. Physiologic dead space is itself normal, but the reduced tidal volume dictates that the dead space to tidal volume ratio is increased: alveolar ventilation is compromised by the *relative* increase in dead space ventilation. Identification of these extrapulmonary mechanisms is dependent upon demonstration of a normal physiologic dead space and a low tidal volume (yielding an elevated dead space to tidal volume ratio) in the presence of normal or low total minute ventilation.

When intrinsic lung disease is present, hypercapnia occurs because of the absolute increase in physiologic dead space that accompanies ventilation/perfusion imbalance. Minute ventilation is usually above normal. Hypercapnia develops when the resultant increase in ventilatory drive is not adequate to compensate for the impaired CO_2 elimination. Minute ventilation may even be low if ventilatory drive is suppressed. Identification of intrapulmonary mechanisms for the hypercapnia is dependent upon demonstration of an absolute increase in calculated physiologic dead space and a high dead space to tidal volume ratio, whether total ventilation and tidal volume are high, normal, or low.

Calculation of physiologic dead space is therefore key in differentiating hypercapnia caused by lung disease from hypercapnia resulting from extrapulmonary mechanisms.

Physiologic Dead Space

The concept of physiologic dead space is analogous to the concept of calculated shunt. Whereas shunt represents the percentage of the *cardiac output* that remains unoxygenated, physiologic dead space represents the percentage of total *ventilation* that does not participate in clearing CO_2 from the lungs. This physiologic dead space results from ventilation to alveolar units that are overventilated relative to perfusion. These $\dot{V}/\dot{Q}$ units range from those with slightly elevated $\dot{V}/\dot{Q}$, to units with essentially infinite $\dot{V}/\dot{Q}$. The concept of physiologic dead space simplifies this variability of $\dot{V}/\dot{Q}$ by considering the lung as being composed of two compartments: one is gas exchanging alveoli; the other is dead space which, by definition, contains no CO_2. In this model, the difference between ideal alveolar PCO_2 and expired PCO_2 is due to dilution of alveolar gas by the dead space volume. Accordingly, the ratio of physiologic dead space to tidal volume is defined by the Bohr dead space equation:

Equation 8-8

$$\frac{V_D}{V_T} = \frac{(\text{Ideal alveolar } PCO_2 - \text{Mixed-expired } PCO_2)}{\text{Ideal alveolar } PCO_2}$$

The mixed-expired PCO_2 can be obtained simply by collecting exhaled gas in a Douglas Bag or mixing chamber and by sampling the gas with a capnograph or mass-spectrometer. The $PaCO_2$ is utilized as a reasonable approximation of ideal $PACO_2$. Since relationships inherent in the Bohr equation assume steady-state conditions, the calculation may be in error if the patient is in a transient state with changing ventilatory levels.

Appendix 8-6 is a series of nomograms that allows one to estimate physiologic dead space to tidal volume ratios from $PaCO_2$ and total minute ventilation. Four nomograms are provided for estimating V_D/V_T at different levels of CO_2 production ranging from 150 ml/min to 300 ml/min. Selection of a nomogram depends upon body size. Assume 100 ml/min/m² CO_2 production in the average sized adult under basal conditions. If clinical judgment suggests that metabolic rate may not be basal, V_D/V_T is more accurately assessed by direct measurement.

EVALUATION OF ACID-BASE BALANCE

The purpose of this section is to review the principles involved in the identification of acid-base disorders from arterial blood gas analysis. Confirmation of the disorder requires the synthesis of information from patient history, clinical examination, plasma and urinary electrolytes, as well as the sequential analysis of acid-base status during development and/or correction of the disorder.

Arterial pH and PCO_2 as well as plasma bicarbonate concentration $[HCO_3{}^-]$ provide the primary tools for the assessment of acid-base status. Arterial blood gas analysis yields pH and PCO_2 by direct measurement. From these parameters, values may be calculated for plasma $[HCO_3{}^-]$ and blood or extracellular base excess.

Acid-base abnormalities can be divided into metabolic and respiratory disorders. Metabolic disorders are caused by the retention or depletion of nonvolatile acids controlled by metabolic processes or renal function, and are reflected in the plasma $[HCO_3{}^-]$. Respiratory disorders result from changes in the volatile $HCO_3{}^-$ − H_2CO_3 system, which is under ventilatory control, and are reflected in the $PaCO_2$. A primary disorder elicits a compensatory response which serves to return the pH toward normal. Compensation alters the ratio of plasma $[HCO_3{}^-]$ to PCO_2, which determines the plasma pH according to the Henderson-Hasselbalch equation (see below).

Hydrogen Ion Activity and pH

Blood gas analyzers measure pH by means of the Severinghaus electrode. This is based upon electrophysical principles that directly equate electrical potential across a glass electrode with hydrogen ion activity. For clinical purposes, hydrogen ion activity and concentration $[H^+]$ are equivalent.[17] Since pH is, by definition, the negative logarithm of $[H^+]$, the pH obtained with the Severinghaus electrode is a measure of plasma acidity.

The interrelationship between pH and hydrogen ion activity is expressed as follows:

Equation 8-9a

$$[H^+] = 10^{(9\text{-pH})}$$

Equation 8-9b

$$pH = -\log\frac{[H^+]}{10^9}$$

Appendix 8-7 provides a nomogram for the precise conversion between these parameters. The nomogram provides a "rule of thumb" for approximating the conversion between pH and $[H^+]$: at pH 7.40 the $[H^+]$ is 40 nEq/l; pH varies inversely with $[H^+]$; a change in pH of 0.01 between pH values 7.20 and 7.50 is roughly equivalent to a change in $[H^+]$ of 1 nEq/l.

The range for normal arterial pH is 7.36–7.44. When $[H^+]$ increases such that arterial pH is lower than 7.36, the blood is considered *acidemic*. Conversely, when hydrogen ion concentration decreases such that arterial pH is greater than 7.44, the blood is considered *alkalemic*. Any process that contributes to an excess of hydrogen ion activity in the body is referred to as an *acidosis; alkalosis* is any process resulting in a whole body deficit of hydrogen ions. The efficiency of the body's buffer systems as well as the secondary compensatory responses determine the degree to which an acidosis or an alkalosis will be reflected in a persisting abnormality of pH (acidemia or alkalemia).

The Henderson-Hasselbalch Equation

The Henderson-Hasselbalch equation[10] represents a logarithmic expression of the dissociation equilibrium of the $HCO_3^- - H_2CO_3$ system. It defines the relationships among pH, PCO_2 (torr), and plasma $[HCO_3^-]$ (mEq/l):

Equation 8-10a

$$pH = pK' + \log\frac{[HCO_3^-]}{(\alpha PCO_2)}$$

It is inherent in this equation that if two variables are known, the third may be calculated. For clinical purposes, the pK' (dissociation constant) is assumed constant at 6.1, and α (solubility coefficient) is 0.03; therefore, the ratio of $[HCO_3^-]$ to αPCO_2 defines pH. For example, at the normal plasma $[HCO_3^-]$ of 24.0 mEq/l and the normal $PaCO_2$ of 40 torr, the ratio is 24.0/1.2 or 20/1. This ratio determines the normal pH of 7.40.

When the ratio of $[HCO_3^-]$ to $\alpha PaCO_2$ increases, the pH rises; when the ratio decreases, the pH falls. Variations in the numerator $[HCO_3^-]$ are predominantly influenced by renal mechanisms; variations in the denominator ($PaCO_2$) reflect changes in carbonic acid (H_2CO_3) and are controlled by respiratory mechanisms.

Plasma Bicarbonate Concentration $[HCO_3^-]$, the Henderson Equation and Total Venous CO_2 Content

The plasma $[HCO_3^-]$ is an essential component of the analysis of acid-base balance. It represents a major extracellular buffer that is readily measured. HCO_3^-

in conjunction with H_2CO_3 accounts for about 40–50 percent of the total-body buffer capacity.

The plasma $[HCO_3^-]$ may be obtained in one of three ways: it may be calculated (from the Henderson-Hasselbalch or the Henderson equations); it may be read from a nomogram (based on a graphic solution of the above equations); or it may be measured in venous blood as total CO_2 content.

Calculation of Plasma Bicarbonate Concentration

The Henderson-Hasselbalch equation provides the basis for calculation of plasma $[HCO_3^-]$. For example, at pH 7.30 and PCO_2 50 torr, the plasma $[HCO_3^-]$ is obtained through substitution in Equation 8-10b.

Equation 8-10b

$$7.30 = 6.1 + \log \frac{[HCO_3^-]}{(0.03 \times 50)}$$

$$7.30 - 6.1 = \log \frac{[HCO_3^-]}{1.5}$$

$$1.20 = \log [HCO_3^-] - \log 1.5$$

$$1.38 = \log [HCO_3^-]$$

$$[HCO_3^-] = \text{antilog } 1.38 = 24.0 \text{ mEq/l}$$

Modern blood gas analyzers provide calculated values for $[HCO_3^-]$ based upon the mathematical relationships implicit in the Henderson-Hasselbalch equation. Alternatively, nomograms provide graphic solutions (Appendices 8-2, 8-8, and 8-9).

The Henderson Equation

The Henderson equation is a nonlogarithmic form of the Henderson-Hasselbalch equation that simplifies calculation.[11] It expresses the relationships among hydrogen ion concentration (nEq/l), PCO_2(torr) and $[HCO_3^-]$ (mEq/l):

Equation 8-11a

$$[H^+] = 24 \times \frac{PCO_2}{[HCO_3^-]}$$

The Henderson equation allows for direct calculation of plasma $[HCO_3^-]$ when both $[H^+]$ and PCO_2 are available. As an example, for pH 7.30 and PCO_2 50 torr, the plasma $[HCO_3^-]$ is obtained by converting the pH to $[H^+]$ and substituting into the Henderson equation. The pH may be converted to $[H^+]$ utilizing Equation 8-9a or the nomogram in Appendix 8-7. The $[H^+]$ may be approximated using a "rule of thumb" (see section on Hydrogen Ion Activity). In the example, the pH of 7.30 is decreased by 0.10 units below a normal pH of 7.40; this is an increase of 10 nEq/l above the normal $[H^+]$ of 40 nEq/l. Thus, pH 7.30 equals a $[H^+]$ of 40 plus 10, or

50 nEq/l. The substitution into the Henderson equation (Equation 8-11a) is as follows:

Equation 8-11b

$$50\ nEq/l = 24 \times \frac{50\ torr}{[HCO_3^-]}$$

$$[HCO_3^-] = 24.0\ mEq/l$$

Total Venous CO₂ Content

The $[HCO_3^-]$ may also be estimated from total venous CO_2 content. The CO_2 content that is standardly reported with venous electrolyte results should be 1 to 3 mEq/l higher than the calculated arterial plasma $[HCO_3^-]$. The difference is accounted for predominantly by dissolved CO_2 in the venous blood. Use of a tourniquet and exercise of the hand may further increase the CO_2 content. It must be recognized that the venous blood is analyzed by a different technique, often in a different laboratory, and that samples may not be simultaneously obtained. Comparison of the venous CO_2 content with the arterial $[HCO_3^-]$ provides a check of the internal consistency of the acid-base parameters; discrepancies between the two identify possible laboratory error, in either the venous or the arterial measurement.

Use of [HCO₃⁻] as an Index of Whole-body Buffer Base

Acid-base disturbances influence whole-body buffering capacity in a predictable manner. Whole-body buffering capacity is composed of interacting buffer systems: the volatile bicarbonate system ($HCO_3^- - H_2CO_3$) and the nonbicarbonate buffers ($Buf^- - HBuf$) consisting predominantly of Hgb, proteins and phosphates. The sum of the buffer anions, HCO_3^- and Buf^-, is the total buffer base that defines total-body buffering capacity.[19] Since all body buffer systems are in equilibrium, a change in the plasma $[HCO_3^-]$ reflects parallel changes in the other body buffer systems if PCO_2 remains constant.

The following equilibrium reaction illustrates the interaction between the $HCO_3^- - H_2CO_3$ buffer system and the other nonbicarbonate buffer systems:

Equation 8-12

$$CO_2 + H_2O \rightleftharpoons H_2CO_3 \rightleftharpoons H^+ + HCO_3^-$$

$$+$$

$$HBuf \rightleftharpoons Buf^-$$

Metabolic acid-base disturbances induce changes in $[H^+]$, which result in the titration of both bicarbonate and nonbicarbonate buffer systems. A change in measured plasma $[HCO_3^-]$ reflects a concomitant change in $[Buf^-]$ in the same direction. Thus, plasma $[HCO_3^-]$ serves as a marker of a change in total buffer anion characteristic of the metabolic component of an acid-base disorder.

The use of the plasma [HCO_3^-] as an index of change in whole-body buffer base is restricted by the fact that the [HCO_3^-] changes with changing PCO_2. In the absence of non-HCO_3^- buffer systems (Buf^-), the dissociation of H_2CO_3 is limited because the H^+ generated is not titrated. In the presence of other buffer systems, H^+ is titrated with Buf^- facilitating the shift of the CO_2 dissociation equilibrium (Equation 8-12) to the right or left as PCO_2 is increased or decreased. Thus, acute changes in PCO_2 result in measurable changes in plasma [HCO_3^-]; [Buf^-] changes in a direction opposite to the [HCO_3^-] as a result of the titration with [H^+]. Accordingly, the change in [HCO_3^-] does not serve as a marker of change in total buffer anion when PCO_2 changes. The interpretation of a change in plasma [HCO_3^-] requires quantitation of the effect of abnormal $PaCO_2$ before being applied to the interpretation of metabolic acid-base disorders.

Standard Bicarbonate and Base Excess (BE)

The calculation of *standard bicarbonate* was designed to quantitate the effect of changing PCO_2 on plasma [HCO_3^-]. The standard [HCO_3^-] represents the [HCO_3^-] if $PaCO_2$ were 40 torr.[13] It is, therefore, a marker of a metabolic acid-base disorder uncomplicated by coincidental changes in [HCO_3^-] due to changes in $PaCO_2$. The concept of *base excess* is an extension of the concept of standard bicarbonate. Blood base excess is an in vitro value that represents the amount of strong acid or base (in mEq/l) that would have to be added to blood equilibrated to a PCO_2 of 40 torr in order to return the pH to 7.40.[10] The blood base excess is equivalent to the difference between the standard bicarbonate concentration and a normal [HCO_3^-] of 24 mEq/l, times a factor that is largely dependent upon hemoglobin concentration. Thus, the blood base excess reflects the deviation of whole-*blood* buffer base from normal, under standard ventilatory conditions.

The clinical application of *blood base excess* is limited since it is based on in vitro relationships. Differences may exist between calculated in vitro and in vivo values due to the dilutional effect of the extravascular compartment, the presence of tissue buffer systems, or a lag in the equilibration of [HCO_3^-] between body compartments.[15] The calculation of *extracellular base excess* was developed to overcome these limitations.[14] An empirically determined [Hgb] of 3–5 Gm percent is assumed for this calculation of base excess to approximate the dilutional effects of extracellular fluid. Extracellular base excess reflects the deviation from normal of whole-*body* buffer base [HCO_3^-] + [Buf^-], under standard ventilatory conditions. The normal range is ± 2 mEq/l; a positive value reflects whole-body base excess, and a negative value reflects base deficit.

The calculation of extracellular base excess quantitates the metabolic component of an acid-base disorder. This quantitation may reflect a primary metabolic disorder or a metabolic compensation to a primary respiratory disorder. It is clinically relevant when $PaCO_2$ is abnormal or when analysis of sequential blood gases reveals changing values for both [HCO_3^-] and $PaCO_2$.

DISORDERS OF ACID-BASE BALANCE

The following sections define the four primary acid-base disorders and illustrate the effect of each disorder on the interacting HCO_3^- and non-HCO_3^- buffer systems.

Respiratory Acidosis

Acute respiratory acidosis is the result of a primary elevation in $PaCO_2$, which leads to the generation of HCO_3^- and H^+ through the dissociation of H_2CO_3. Equation 8-12 illustrates the interacting buffer systems. In respiratory acidosis, total-body buffer anion ([HCO_3^-] + [Buf^-] remains constant. Arterial blood gas analysis reveals acidemia and increased PCO_2 along with a small but predictable increase in plasma [HCO_3^-] that approximates 1 mEq/l per 10 torr increase in PCO_2. This increase in [HCO_3^-] is dependent on the presence of the non-bicarbonate buffer systems (HBuf). The titration of H^+ by Buf^- shifts the CO_2 equilibrium to the right, increasing [HCO_3^-]. The increase in plasma [HCO_3^-] will be counterbalanced by an equivalent decrease in [Buf^-] as H^+ is titrated to HBuf. The sum of [HCO_3^-] and [Buf^-] will remain unchanged. Since total buffer anion remains constant, the calculated extracellular base excess remains unchanged with acute respiratory acidosis despite the increased plasma [HCO_3^-].

Chronic respiratory acidosis is identified by the presence of a metabolic adjustment for the primary respiratory disturbance. When respiratory acidosis is sustained, retention of HCO_3^- results from the renal compensatory response. The increase of [HCO_3^-] shifts the HCO_3^- − H_2CO_3 equilibrium back toward normal; [H^+] remains elevated to the degree that compensation is not complete. The non-HCO_3^- buffer system remains titrated in favor of HBuf. Despite the reduction in [Buf^-], the added HCO_3^- results in an increase in whole-body buffer base. The sum of [HCO_3^-] and [Buf^-], and therefore, calculated extracellular base excess, increases. This base excess reflects the compensatory response and does not imply a primary metabolic abnormality. The compensatory response is seldom complete and results in a degree of persisting acidemia that varies with the chronic $PaCO_2$ level.

Respiratory Alkalosis

Acute respiratory alkalosis is the result of a primary decrease in $PaCO_2$, which leads to a decrease in [HCO_3^-] and [H^+] through a shift of the CO_2 equilibrium to the left, and decreased dissociation of H_2CO_3.

Arterial blood gas analysis reveals alkalemia and decreased $PaCO_2$ associated with a small and predictable decrease in plasma [HCO_3^-] that approximates 2 mEq/l per 10 torr decrease in PCO_2. This decrease in [HCO_3^-] is dependent on the presence of non-bicarbonate buffer systems (HBuf), which allow the CO_2 equilibrium to shift to the left by releasing H^+. The decrease in plasma [HCO_3^-] will be counterbalanced by an equivalent increase in [Buf^-]. As in acute respiratory acidosis, the sum of $[HCO_3^-]$ and $[Buf^-]$ will remain unchanged, and the calculated extracellular base excess will not decrease.

Chronic respiratory alkalosis is identified by the presence of a metabolic adjustment for the primary respiratory disturbance. When respiratory alkalosis is sustained, net loss of HCO_3^- results from the renal compensatory response. The decrease of $[HCO_3^-]$ shifts the $HCO_3^- - H_2CO_3$ equilibrium back toward normal; $[H^+]$ remains depressed to the degree that compensation is not complete. The non-HCO_3^- buffer system remains titrated toward Buf^-. Despite the increase in $[Buf^-]$, the lost HCO_3^- results in a decrease in whole-body buffer base ($[HCO_3^-]$ + $[Buf^-]$). This decreased base excess (base deficit) reflects the compensatory response and does not imply a primary metabolic abnormality. The compensatory response is seldom complete and results in a degree of persisting alkalemia that varies with the chronic $PaCO_2$ level.

The terms "acute" and "chronic" as applied to respiratory acid-base disorders are synonymous with "uncompensated" or "compensated" and do not necessarily imply duration of the disorder. The renal response is immediate but may not be measurable or fully reflected in the plasma $[HCO_3^-]$ for several days.

Metabolic Acidosis

Metabolic acidosis is defined as an accumulation of H^+ or loss of base resulting in a decrease in whole-body buffer base. The addition of acid or loss of base from the body results in a net increase of H^+, which influences all buffer systems. The resulting increase in $[H^+]$ shifts the CO_2 equilibrium to the left, (Equation 8-12) reducing $[HCO_3^-]$ and transiently increasing $PaCO_2$; concomitantly, the H^+ titrates Buf^- to $HBuf$. Thus, buffer anion $[HCO_3^-]$ + $[Buf^-]$ is decreased, reflecting a decrease in total body buffer base.

Arterial blood gas analysis reveals the expected acidemia with reduction of both $[HCO_3^-]$ and extracellular base excess (base deficit). The increase in $PaCO_2$ dictated by the shift of the CO_2 equilibrium to the left is transient and is not seen clinically for two reasons: CO_2 is volatile and is released from the lungs; the acidemia is an immediate stimulus for increased ventilation which then decreases the $PaCO_2$ below normal. The reduction in PCO_2 is the compensation which returns the pH toward normal.

Metabolic acidosis may be due to the accumulation of organic or inorganic acids. The anion gap is a helpful tool in suggesting the presence and clarifying the differential diagnosis of a metabolic acidosis. The numerical difference between Na^+, the measured cation, and HCO_3^- + Cl^-, the measured anions, reflects unmeasured anions. This difference normally approximates 8–12 mEq/l:

Equation 8-13

$$\text{Anion gap (mEq/l)} = [Na^+] - ([HCO_3^-] + [Cl^-])$$

When metabolic acidosis is due to the accumulation of organic acids, as in diabetic ketoacidosis, the reduced HCO_3^- is replaced by the organic anion that is not measured. The Na^+ is counterbalanced by HCO_3^-, Cl^-, and the unmeasured anion. Thus, the anion gap calculated from standard venous electrolytes will increase. Metabolic acidosis of gastrointestinal or renal origin is due to the accumulation of inorganic acid, usually HCl. In this circumstance, the anion gap remains normal since the decrease in plasma $[HCO_3^-]$ is counterbalanced by the increase in plasma $[Cl^-]$.

Metabolic Alkalosis

Metabolic alkalosis results from an increase in base or loss of acid resulting in an increase in whole-body buffer base. The increase of $[HCO_3^-]$ shifts the CO_2 equilibrium to the left, decreasing $[H^+]$ and transiently increasing $PaCO_2$; concomitantly, the decrease in $[H^+]$ induces dissociation of HBuf, increasing $[Buf^-]$. Thus, buffer anion ($[HCO_3^-]$ + $[Buf^-]$) is increased, reflecting an increase in total body buffer base.

Arterial blood gas analysis reveals the expected alkalemia, increased $[HCO_3^-]$, and extracellular base excess. The increase in $PaCO_2$ dictated by the shift of the CO_2 equilibrium to the left is sustained by a decrease in ventilation in response to the alkalemia. The magnitude of this respiratory response to metabolic alkalosis is smaller and less predictable than in metabolic acidosis. Compensatory increase in $PaCO_2$ helps return arterial pH toward normal.

The terms "acute" and "chronic" as applied to a metabolic acid-base disorder usually do imply duration of the disorder. Acute metabolic acidosis or alkalosis implies a transient state; chronic metabolic acidosis implies a steady-state. The respiratory compensation is immediately demonstrated by changes in $PaCO_2$ although it may not be complete for hours until body compartments reach equilibrium.

IDENTIFICATION OF ACID-BASE DISORDERS

Table 8-3 summarizes the four primary acid-base disturbances. Metabolic disorders are characterized by a change in $[HCO_3^-]$ reflecting a change in total body base; metabolic acidosis results in low $[HCO_3^-]$ and low pH; metabolic alkalosis

Table 8-3
Primary Acid-Base Disturbances

Primary Disorder	Initial Abnormality	Compensatory Response
Metabolic acidosis	Decreased pH, Decreased $[HCO_3^-]$ Base deficit	Decreased $PaCO_2$
Metabolic alkalosis	Increased pH, Increased $[HCO_3^-]$ Base excess	Increased $PaCO_2$
Respiratory acidosis	Decreased pH, Increased $PaCO_2$	Increased HCO_3^- Base excess
Respiratory alkalosis	Increased pH, Decreased $PaCO_2$	Decreased HCO_3^- Base deficit

results in elevated $[HCO_3^-]$ and high pH. Compensation is via the respiratory system and is reflected in alteration of $PaCO_2$, which returns the pH toward normal. Respiratory disorders alter the $PaCO_2$; respiratory acidosis is characterized by elevated $PaCO_2$ and low pH; respiratory alkalosis is characterized by reduced $PaCO_2$ levels and high pH. Compensation is via the kidney and is reflected in changes of plasma $[HCO_3^-]$. The primary disorder (acidosis or alkalosis) is identified by an abnormal plasma $[HCO_3^-]$ and/or $PaCO_2$; plasma pH is usually abnormal (acidemia or alkalemia), with the degree of abnormality depending on the degree of compensation.

Mixed-disorders involve two or more underlying primary disturbances and are conceptually distinct from compensated simple disorders. The distinction between compensation and a second primary acid-base disorder is essential in defining therapeutic goals. Therapy directed to a primary disorder will result in spontaneous reversal of compensatory changes. Two therapeutic approaches need to be considered if two primary disorders coexist. These distinctions may be difficult to make initially and may depend on serial observations during the course of the illness.

Nomograms and Regression Formulae

The patterns of compensation for each of the acid-base disorders have been defined empirically. Studies in animals and man during induced or spontaneous disturbances have shown that the degree of compensation follows predictable patterns which vary with the magnitude of the primary disturbance. These patterns are expressed graphically as nomograms and mathematically as regression equations.[12,15,17,18,20]

These nomograms and equations provide a framework for the evaluation of acid-base abnormality from arterial blood gas analysis.

The acid-base nomograms have been published in various forms. Two versions are presented (Appendix 8-8 and 8-9). These nomograms have in common, coordinates and isopleths based on a graphic solution of the Hendersen-Hasselbalch equation. Appendix 8-8 utilizes as coordinates the markers of whole-body response to acid-base disorder, plasma $[HCO_3^-]$, and PCO_2. Both nomograms superimpose confidence bands depicting the empirically determined compensatory responses to each of the primary acid-base disorders. These responses are expressed as regression formulae in Table 8-4.

The nomograms allow for comparison of observed data with values predicted for each primary acid-base disorder and suggest whether they are in accord with a simple or a mixed disorder. The blood gas values are consistent with a simple acid-base disorder when the point representing the observed values falls within the 95 percent confidence band of that disorder (or agrees with values predicted by the relevant regression formula). If the point falls outside the defined confidence band for a simple disorder, this suggests that either a transient state or a mixed abnormality is present. The confidence bands serve as guides to clinical interpretation and do not confirm an acid-base disturbance until the patient's overall clinical picture warrants this judgment.

Table 8-4
Formulas for Predicting Compensatory Responses for Acid-Base Disturbances

Respiratory Acidosis	Reference
Acute:	
Expected $\Delta [H^+] = 0.75 \times \Delta PaCO_2$	12
$[HCO_3^-]$ increases 1 mEq/l for every 10 torr increase in $PaCO_2$	17
Chronic:	
Expected $\Delta [H^+] = 0.30 \times \Delta PaCO_2$	12
$[HCO_3^-]$ increases 3.5 mEq/l for every 10 torr increase in $PaCO_2$	17
Respiratory Alkalosis	
Acute:	
Expected $\Delta [H^+] = 0.75 \times \Delta PaCO_2$	12
$[HCO_3^-]$ decreases 2 mEq/l for every 10 torr in $PaCO_2$	17
Chronic:	
Expected $\Delta [H^+] = 0.17 \times \Delta PaCO_2$	17
$[HCO_3^-]$ decreases 5 mEq/l for every 10 torr decrease in $PaCO_2$	17
Metabolic Acidosis	
Expected $PaCO_2 = 1.5 \times$ Measured $[HCO_3^-] + 8 \pm 2$	16
Expected $\Delta PaCO_2 = 1.2 \times \Delta [HCO_3^-]$	12
Metabolic Alkalosis	
Expected $PaCO_2 = 0.9 \times$ Measured $[HCO_3^-] + 9$	17
Expected $\Delta PaCO_2 = 0.7 \times \Delta [HCO_3^-]$	12

The confidence bands in the acid-base nomograms (Appendix 8-8 and 8-9) do not incorporate the calculation of base excess; the expected whole-body response for each acid-base disorder is expressed in terms of $HCO_3^- - PCO_2$ or $pH - PCO_2$ relationships. The calculation of base excess supplements the use of the nomograms by quantitating the metabolic component independent of changing $PaCO_2$.

Clinical Examples

Metabolic Acidosis

Venous total CO_2 content is reduced at 13.2 mEq/l suggesting a total-body base deficit (Table 8-5). Arterial blood gas analysis reveals a pH of 7.29 and PCO_2 of 25 torr. Pattern analysis is consistent with metabolic acidosis with partial respiratory compensation (see Table 8-3). Arterial plasma $[HCO_3^-]$ may be read from Appendix 8-2 or calculated through substitution in the Hendersen equation:

Table 8-5
Clinical Example 1: Diabetic Ketoacidosis

Arterial Blood Gas:		Venous Electrolytes:			
pH	PCO_2 (torr)	$[Na^+]$ (mEq/L)	$[K^+]$ (mEq/L)	$[CO_2]$ (mEq/L)	$[Cl^-]$ (mEq/L)
7.29	25	133	4.0	13.2	102

Step 1: (Equation 8-9a or read from Appendix 8-7).

$$[H^+] = 10^{(9-7.29)} = 51 \text{ nEq/l}$$

Step 2: (Substitution in Equation 8-11)

$$51 = 24 \times \frac{25}{[HCO_3^-]}$$

$$[HCO_3^-] = 12 \text{ mEq/l}$$

This reduced arterial plasma $[HCO_3^-]$ of 12 mEq/l agrees with the venous total CO_2 content of 13.2 mEq/l and confirms the arterial and venous values. The extracellular base excess (read from Appendix 8-2) of -14 mEq/l confirms and quantitates the base deficit.

Blood gas values plotted on either acid-base nomogram (Appendix 8-8 or 8-9) fall within the confidence band for metabolic acidosis. This is in accord with a simple disorder and indicates that the degree of compensation ($\Delta PaCO_2$) is appropriate for this degree of acidosis (as reflected in the $\Delta[HCO_3^-]$.

Alternatively, blood gas values may be compared to the confidence band for metabolic acidosis through substitution in a regression equation (Table 8-4):

$$\Delta PaCO_2 = 1.2 \times (24 - 14) = 12 \text{ torr}$$

Thus, the $PaCO_2$ expected for this degree of metabolic acidosis is approximately $(40 - 12)$ or 28 torr, which is similar to the observed $PaCO_2$ of 25 torr.

The use of calculated base deficit supplements these conclusions by quantitating the degree of metabolic acidosis and provides a method for following the metabolic component of the disorder as $[HCO_3^-]$ and $PaCO_2$ both change.

Calculation of the anion gap through substitution of values for $[Na^+]$, $[Cl^-]$, and $[HCO_3^-]$ in Equation 8-13 indicates the presence of unmeasured anion:

$$\text{Anion Gap} = 133 - (102 + 13.2)$$
$$= 17.8 \text{ (mEq/l)}$$

The patient in this example has a history of Diabetes Mellitus, which suggests ketoacidosis as a likely cause for the acid-base abnormality. The increased anion gap is consistent with diabetic ketoacidosis.

Mixed Respiratory Acidosis and Metabolic Alkalosis

Venous total CO_2 content (Table 8-6A) is increased at 44.0 mEq/l suggesting a total-body base excess. Arterial blood gas analysis reveals increased values for pH (7.45) and $PaCO_2$ (60 torr). Pattern analysis suggests metabolic alkalosis since the increased CO_2 content coexists with an elevation in arterial pH (Table 8-3). The increased arterial plasma $[HCO_3^-]$ of 42.3 mEq/l (read from Appendix 8-2 or calculated through substitution in the Henderson equation) is in accord with the

Table 8-6
Clinical Example 2A: CAO and Cor Pulmonale, Intensive Diuretic Therapy
2B: Diuretics Discontinued, KCL Replacement

| Arterial Blood Gas: | | | Extracellular | Venous Electrolytes: | | | |
pH	PCO$_2$ (torr)	[HCO$_3$$^-$] (mEq/l)	Base Excess (mEq/l)	[Na$^+$] (mEq/l)	[K$^+$] (mEq/l)	[CO$_2$] (mEq/l)	[Cl$^-$] (mEq/l)
2A: 7.45	60	42.3	16.6	140	3.5	44.0	88
2B: 7.37	54	31.4	5.6	141	4.5	33.0	100

venous total CO_2 content of 44.0 mEq/l. The extracellular base excess (read from Appendix 8-2) of 16.6 mEq/l confirms and quantitates the total-body base excess.

Whereas the elevated base excess in this example quantifies the metabolic component of the acid-base disorder, it does not distinguish between metabolic alkalosis and metabolic compensation for a primary respiratory disorder.

Blood gas values plotted on either acid-base nomogram (Appendix 8-8 or 8-9) do not fall within the range for a simple disorder but are midway between the confidence band for metabolic alkalosis and chronic respiratory acidosis, implying that the disorder is mixed.

The patient in this example has a history of CAO, has received intensive diuretic therapy, and is hypochloremic with a $[Cl^-]$ of 88 mEq/l.

Table 8-6B includes clinical data after diuretic therapy has been discontinued and KCl replacement given. The $[K^+]$ and $[Cl^-]$ have returned to normal levels. Venous CO_2 has decreased from 44.0 to 33.0 mEq/l, remaining elevated.

Arterial blood gas analysis now demonstrates borderline acidemia, with a pH that has decreased from 7.45 to 7.37, and persistent hypercapnia, with a $PaCO_2$ that has decreased from 60 to 54 torr. The calculated arterial $[HCO_3^-]$ is 31.4 mEq/l and is in accord with the venous CO_2 content.

Pattern analysis is consistent with a compensated respiratory acidosis since a nearly normal pH coexists with an elevated $[HCO_3^-]$ and $PaCO_2$. This is confirmed by plotting the values on an acid-base map (Appendix 8-8 or 8-9): the point now falls within the confidence band for chronic respiratory acidosis.

The extracellular base excess has decreased from 16.6 to 5.6 mEq/l quantitating the metabolic response to treatment. This change in base excess corresponds to the change in plasma $[HCO_3^-]$ since the change in $PaCO_2$ is small. The residual abnormality in $[HCO_3^-]$ and base excess reflects the metabolic compensation to the underlying respiratory acidosis.

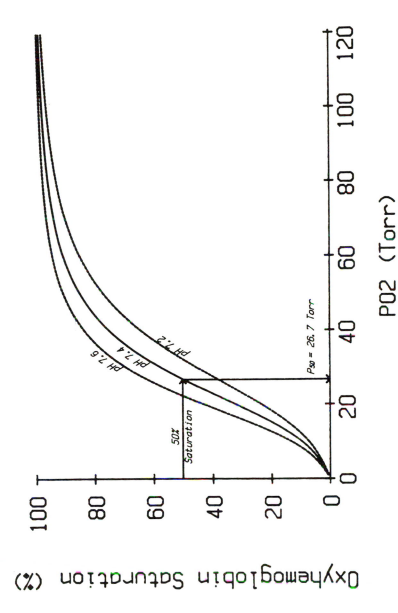

Appendix 8-1. Oxyhemoglobin dissociation curve (hemoglobin A) at various pH values. The standard P_{50} is indicated.

117

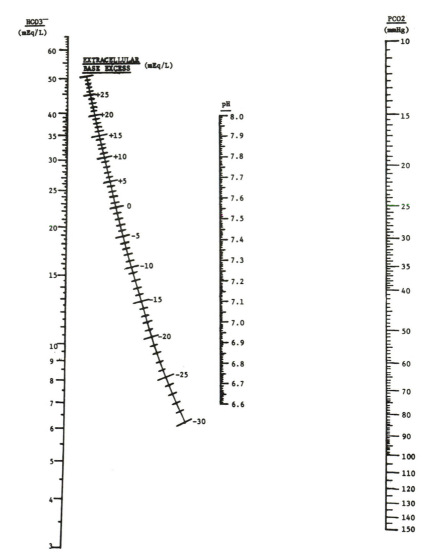

Appendix 8-2. Acid Base Alignment Nomogram. Values for plasma bicarbonate concentration and extracellular base excess may be obtained by extending a line drawn through the measured pH and PCO₂. (Revised from Siggaard-Andersen[1], with permission.)

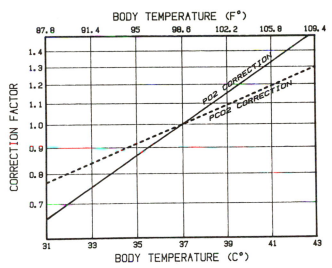

Appendix 8-3. Nomogram for correction of PO_2 and PCO_2 from temperature of blood gas analyzer (37°) to patient's body temperature. Read PO_2 or PCO_2 correction factor at patient's body temperature and multiply by measured PO_2 or PCO_2. (Correction for PO_2 from Severinghaus[3]; for PCO_2 from Kelman and Nunn[2].)

SHUNT NOMOGRAM

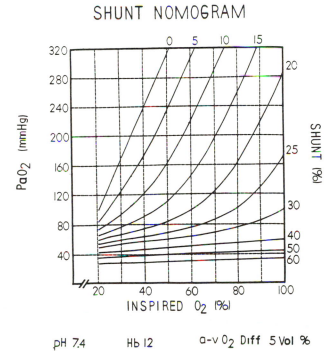

pH 7.4　　　Hb 12　　　a-v O_2 Diff 5 Vol %

Appendix 8-4. Nomogram for estimating shunt at various FIO_2 levels. This is applicable when cardiac output is normal. Variations in pH and [Hgb] from the values assumed in the nomogram do not have as great an effect on the accuracy of this nomogram.

119

SHUNT NOMOGRAM

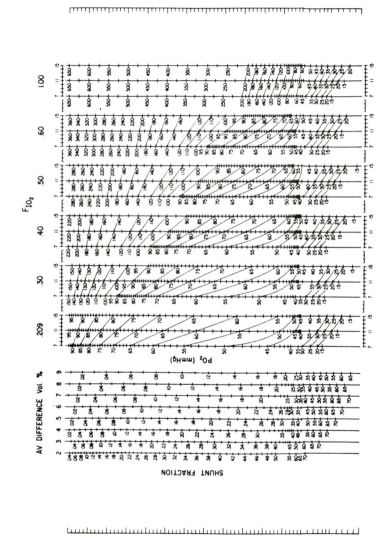

Appendix 8-5. Nomogram for estimating shunt at various FIO₂ levels. This is applicable when cardiac output and/or [Hgb] are abnormal. Instructions for use: draw a horizontal line through the measured PO₂ in the column below the most appropriate FIO₂ and Hgb headings; read the shunt fraction below the measured (or assumed) AV difference. (Revised from Shapiro and Peters[9], with permission)

DEAD SPACE NOMOGRAMS

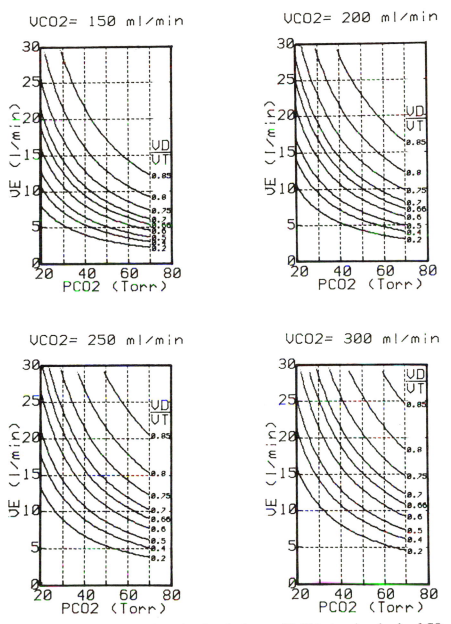

Appendix 8-6. Nomograms for estimating dead space (V_D/V_T) at various levels of CO_2 production. Select the appropriate nomogram by assuming basal CO_2 production equals 100 ml/min/m².

CONVERSION OF pH TO [H+]

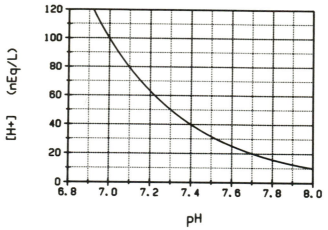

Appendix 8-7. Nomogram for Conversion of pH to [H$^+$] in nEq/l. Note that for pH 7.30 — 7.50 a pH change of 0.01 units is roughly equivalent to a change in [H$^+$] of 1 nEq/l.

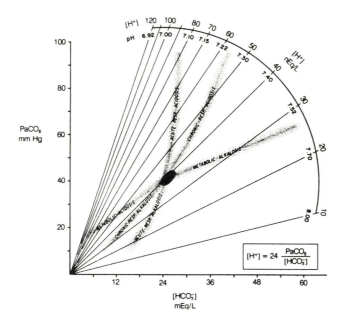

Appendix 8-8. Nomogram utilizing a graphic solution of the Henderson-Hasselbalch equation to characterize acid-base disorders. Confidence bands representing the acute and chronic primary acid-base disorders are superimposed. This graph utilizes the markers of whole-body response to acid-base disorder (plasma [HCO$_3$$^-$] and PaCO$_2$) to define the X and Y coordinates. (From Cohen and Kassirer[12].)

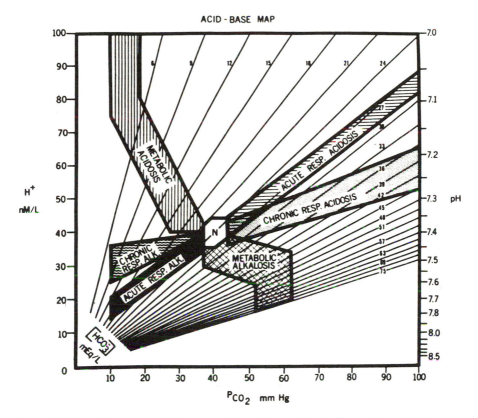

Appendix 8-9. Nomogram utilizing a graphic solution of the Hendersen-Hasselbalch equation to characterize acid-base disorders. Confidence bands representing the acute and chronic primary acid-base disorders are superimposed. This graph utilizes the measured arterial blood gas values (pH and PCO_2) to define the X and Y coordinates. (From Goldberg, et. al.[18].)

References

1. Siggaard-Andersen O. Blood acid-base alignment nomogram. Scand J Clin Lab Invest 15:211–217, 1963
2. Kelman GR, Nunn JF. Nomograms for correction of blood PO_2, PCO_2, pH, and base excess for time and temperature. J Appl Physiol 21:1484–1490, 1966
3. Severinghaus JW. Simple, accurate equations for human blood O_2 dissociation computations, J Appl Physiol 46:599–602, 1979
4. Riley RL, Cournand A. "Ideal" alveolar air and the analysis of ventilation/perfusion relationships in the lungs, J Appl Physiol 1:825–847, 1949
5. Shapiro BA, Harrison RA, Trout CA. Clinical Application of Blood Gases (ed 2). Chicago, YearBook Medical Publishers, 1977

6. Gilbert R, Auchincloss JR, Kuppinger M., et al. Stability of the arterial/alveolar oxygen partial pressure ratio—effects of low ventilation/perfusion regions. Crit Care Med 7:267–272, 1979

7. Kelman GR, Nunn JF. Computer Produced Physiological Tables. New York, Appleton-Century-Crofts, 1968, p 49

8. West JB, Wagner PD. Lung Biology in Health and Disease: Bioengineering Aspects of the Lung. New York, Marcel Dekker Inc., 1977, p 361

9. Shapiro AR, Peters RM. A nomogram for planning respiratory therapy. Chest 72:197, 1977

10. Davenport HW. The ABC of Acid-Base Chemistry (ed 5). Chicago, The University of Chicago Press, 1969

11. Kassirer JP, Bleich HL. Rapid estimation of plasma carbon dioxide from pH and total carbon dioxide content. N Engl J Med 272:1067, 1965

12. Cohen JJ, Kassirer JP. Acid-Base. Boston, Little, Brown and Co, 1982

13. Astrup P, Jorgensen K, Siggaard Andersen O, et al. Acid-base metabolism—New approach. Lancet 1:1035–1039, 1960

14. Severinghaus JW. Acid-base balance nomogram—a Boston-Copenhagen detente. Anesth 48:539, 1976

15. Schwartz WB, Relman AS. A critique of the parameters used in the evaluation of acid-base disorders. "Whole-Blood Buffer Base" and "Standard Bicarbonate" compared with blood pH and plasma bicarbonate concentration. N Engl J Med 268:1382, 1963

16. Albert MD, Dell RB, Winters RW. Quantitative displacement of acid-base equilibrium in metabolic acidosis. Ann Intern Med 66:312, 1967

17. Narins RG, Emmett M. Simple and mixed acid-base disorders—a practical approach. Med 59:161, 1980

18. Goldberg M, Green SB, Moss ML, et al. Computer-based instruction and diagnosis of acid-base disorders. JAMA 223:269, 1973

19. Singer RB, Hastings AB. Improved clinical method for estimation of disturbances of acid-base balance of human blood. Medicine 27:223, 1948

20. Siggaard-Andersen O. An acid-base chart for arterial blood with normal and pathophysiological reference areas. Scand J Clin Lab Invest 27:239, 1971

Part III

Reporting Test Results

9

Prediction Equations and "Normal Values" for Pulmonary Function Tests

Albert Miller

Regression Equations
The Age Variable
The Smoking Variable
  Spirometry and flows
  D_LCO_{SB}
  Usefulness of a smoking coefficient
Race
Which values to call abnormal?
  Conventional Definitions of the lower limits of normal
    Percentage of predicted value
    Ratios to lung volume
  Statistical Definitions of the lower limits of normal
    The need for a statistically valid definition of abnormal
    The fifth percentile
    The 95% confidence interval
Quantitation of Abnormality
Which Prediction Equations to Use?
  Spirometry (FVC, FEV_1), Mean ($FEF_{25-75\%}$) and Instantaneous
    ($FEF_{50\%}$ and $FEF_{75\%}$) Maximum Flows
  Single Breath Diffusing Capacity (D_LCO_{SB})
  Maximum Voluntary Ventilation
  Total Lung Capacity, Functional Residual Capacity, and Residual Volume
  Peak Flow Rate (PFR)
  Maximum Respiratory Pressures

PULMONARY FUNCTION TESTS: A   ISBN 0-8089-1764-4   Copyright © 1987 by Grune & Stratton
GUIDE FOR THE STUDENT AND HOUSE OFFICER

REGRESSION EQUATIONS

The   st we are measuring (e.g., FVC) is called the *dependent variable*. A *regression equation* relates the mean value of the dependent variable in a population to different *independent* variables. It allows us to calculate the expected value of the dependent variable (the test in which we are interested) from knowledge of these *predictor* values.

Age and height are the most widely used independent variables for pulmonary function measurements. Others may be weight, body surface area, hemoglobin concentration (for D_L), or smoking. Simple linear equations using height and age predict spirometric parameters in adults as well as do complex nonlinear models.

The variability of observations about the regression equation is expressed as the *standard deviation* of the equation (SD, Sy.x or standard error of the estimate [SEE]). This reflects the variability of the instruments and recording system, the variability within each individual, and the inherent biologic variation from individual to individual in the function measured. The variability of flow rates is greater than the variability of VC or FEV_1.

THE AGE VARIABLE

All pulmonary function tests (except RV and TLC) decline with age. There is increasing evidence that FVC and FEV_1 plateau after reaching a maximum value in early adulthood, and start to decline between 25 and 35 years of age. The increase in early life is not explained entirely by growth in height. Greater muscle strength plays a role as well. (See Chapter 2).

THE SMOKING VARIABLE

Spirometry and Flows

Current cigarette smokers have lower values for these measurements even if they are clinically "normal." Exsmokers are generally intermediate. Analysis of *asymptomatic* subjects in Michigan revealed significant differences in FEV_1 and flows in male smokers.[1] When subjects who had symptoms attributable to smoking, such as cough and sputum, were studied, differences in the measurements were noted in females (as well as differences in FVC in both sexes). The most useful smoking variable was duration: the coefficient for FEV_1 in normal males was 0.094 L/decade of smoking or 40 percent of the effect of aging.

D_LCO_{SB}

We have published[2] smoking coefficients that account for the 15–25% difference in this test between normal smokers and nonsmokers.

Usefulness of a Smoking Coefficient

It must be understood that the harmful effects of smoking on lung function cannot be detected by statistical analysis of *mean* data alone. Only a small proportion of smokers will develop disabling disease. Their accelerated loss of function will be obscured by the smaller decrements in the vast majority. As Fletcher[3] put it, "The mean value . . . is not the best index for comparing the effects of smoking . . . for the effect on the susceptible minority tends to be overwhelmed by the unaffected majority."

Quantitation of the smoking variable allows the effects of smoking to be separated from the effects of normal aging on the one hand and from the effects of *other* noxious inhalants or diseases on the other. Such an approach is valuable in analyzing the pulmonary function results of patients with clinically diagnosed lung diseases who also smoke.

RACE

Values for TLC, FVC, FEV_1 and flows are scaled down by 13 percent, while values for FRC and RV are reduced by 8 percent when regression equations derived from white populations are used for black subjects.[4] Another way of saying this is that the height coefficients are smaller probably; this probably reflects a smaller proportion of total height contributed by the trunk. There are no differences in D_LCO_{SB} reported between black and white subjects but the matter has not been sufficiently studied.

It remains undetermined whether there are differences among white subjects of different nationalities.

WHICH VALUES TO CALL ABNORMAL?

Conventional Definitions of the Lower Limits of Normal

Percentage of Predicted Value

The conventional rule of thumb has been to classify values for VC, FEV_1, MVV, RV, and TLC less than 80 percent of predicted (or greater than 120 percent of predicted for *increased* RV) as abnormal. For MMF and D_LCO_{SB}, many laboratories consider values less than 75 percent of predicted to be abnormal.

Ratios to Lung Volumes

To FVC (or VC): FEV. Studies by many investigators during the 1950s demonstrated that 95 percent of normal subjects exhale >75 percent of their FVC within the first second. Within the first 0.75 second, the percentage of FVC expired is 70 and within the first 0.5 second, 58.[5] Thus, for many years, 0.75 was considered the lower limit of normal for FEV_1/FVC. Recent practice has been to use 0.70 as the cut-off value; however, FEV_1/FVC falls both with increasing age and with increasing height. This renders use of a constant value for all subjects invalid.

For advanced ages (> 55 and especially > 70 years), FVC tends to decline more than FEV_1 and the FEV_1/FVC will rise.

There is evidence[6,7] that athletes and others whose work activities develop the pectoral muscles (including the accessory muscles of respiration[8]), have a relatively greater than normal FVC compared to FEV_1, with a resulting lower FEV_1/FVC.

Because the FVC is reduced more than the slow or inspired VC in patients with severe airways obstruction with air trapping, the FEV_1/FVC ratio is sometimes misleadingly high in these patients.

MMF. The MMF/FVC ratio has been used to classify patients as to restrictive (> 0.80) or obstructive (< 0.45) impairment;[9] a lower limit of 0.65 has been proposed.[10,11] This permits rapid assessment of the significance of a reported value for MMF when the FVC is reduced.

Equation 9.1

$$\frac{MMF}{FVC} = \frac{1}{2\ MET}$$

Stated another way, MMF/FVC is the reciprocal of twice the MET. Since the MET can be obtained from the MMF and the FVC, it is simpler to use the MET as a flow-related measurement, which is independent of volume and has an upper limit of normal of 0.77 (equivalent to an MMF/FVC ratio of 0.65).

Instantaneous flows. Such flows are sometimes reported as a ratio to FVC. Whether their considerable variability is reduced by this approach is not agreed upon. When evaluating an MEVF curve, it is easy to remember that $FEF_{50\%}/FVC$ should be about 1.0 and $FEF_{75\%}/FVC$ about 0.5 in normal subjects.

Closing volume. This is reported relative to VC; the ratio increases with age.

To TLC: Residual volume, D_L, and closing capacity are often reported as a ratio to TLC. When reported in this way, they are usually designated "specific," e.g., "specific $D_L CO_{SB}$."

Statistical Definitions of the Lower Limits of Normal

The Need for a Statistically Valid Definition of Abnormal

A rational statistical basis for the conventional "80 percent of predicted" rule does not exist. It is true that for the FVC and FEV_1 in *certain* series, a value that is 80 percent of predicted has a confidence approximating 95 percent for subjects who happen to be near the mean age and height of the normal population tested. This is not true for subjects at different ages and heights.

Fig. 9-1. The relationships between the regression line for FVC (males) at a height of 70 inches (slightly modified from Morris[15]), the line for 80 percent of predicted, and the line for 95 percent confidence. The line for 80 percent of predicted approaches the regression line while the line for the 95 percent confidence lower limit is at a constant interval from the regression. [From Miller A, Thornton JC. The interpretation of spirometric measurements in epidemiologic surveys. Environ Res 23:454, 1980, with permission.]

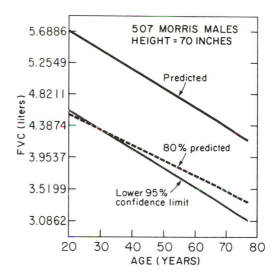

Use of 80 percent of predicted as the lower limit of normal, especially for flow rates, will lead to the identification as abnormal of many subjects whose values are within 95 percent confidence limits, particularly when they are shorter or older. On the other hand, the values for FVC and FEV_1 for taller and younger subjects may erroneously be considered "normal" because they are > 80 percent predicted when in fact they are below the 95 percent confidence limits. This is illustrated by Figures 9-1 and 9-2, which show the relationship between the regression line for FVC and

Fig. 9-2. The relationships between the regression line for FEV_1 in L (versus height, right panel) and $FEF_{25-75\%}$ in L/sec (versus age, left panel), the line for 80 percent of predicted and the line for the 95 percent confidence lower limit. For FEV_1, the relationships are similar to those for FVC regressed against age in Figure 9-1, since smaller values are to the right. For $FEF_{25-75\%}$, use of 80 percent of predicted classifies more subjects as abnormal than does the statistical definition at all ages but the difference between the two lines is greater with smaller values (greater age). [From Sobol BJ. The early detection of airway obstruction: Another perspective. Am J Med 60:623, 1976, with permission.]

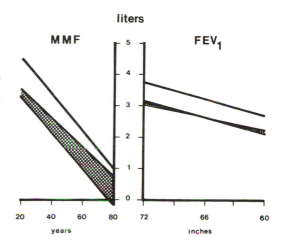

FEV$_1$ (respectively), the line for 80 percent of predicted, and the line for the 95 percent confidence lower limit.

For flows, which have greater variability than FVC or FEV$_1$, it is seen that values below the conventional cut-off (either 75 percent or 80 percent) may be classified as abnormal *at all ages* even though they are above the 95 percent confidence lower limit. Because the statistically defined confidence interval is relatively constant, while the percentage of predicted interval becomes smaller as the predicted value becomes smaller, the likelihood that a value will be "falsely" classified as abnormal is greater at greater age (or lesser height, etc.).

The Fifth Percentile (also called the "Normal 95th Percentile")

The values from the survey population are adjusted for age and height and ordered numerically. That value that divides the 95 percent of the population with the better (generally, larger) values from the 5 percent with the poorer (lower) values is used to separate normal from abnormal. Since values of pulmonary function tests are distributed more-or-less symmetrically about the regression line for age (i.e., at each decade of age the distribution of values is Gaussian) and since the distribution of residuals (predicted value-observed value) is Gaussian, percentile ranking is equivalent to the lower 95 percent confidence interval discussed in the next section.

When the distribution of values is not symmetrical, the percentile method is preferred.[12] In addition, the fifth percentile may be a more practical way to define abnormality when variability is great, as for flow rates. The lower 95 percent confidence limit is then quite low and may even be less than zero when the predicted value is small, as in older subjects. It thus defines a range where no values can exist.

The 95 Percent Confidence Interval (95 Percent Prediction Interval)

This definition of normal can be applied because, for most pulmonary function tests, the values are normally distributed around the regression line with uniform variance. (The term for this is homoscedastic: the scatter is as wide at smaller values as at larger.)

In evaluating most pulmonary function abnormalities, we are concerned only with values at the lower end of the distribution curve, (i.e., we are interested in a one-sided distribution). The *lower* 95 percent confidence interval can be estimated for a one-sided distribution by subtracting 1.645 X SEE (standard error of the estimate) from the predicted value (in L, L/sec, etc.). The SEE (or SD of the equation or Sy.x) is included with the equation when it is published. Since 1.645 X SEE is a constant, this value is simply subtracted from the predicted value to arrive at the 95 percent confidence lower limit. Thus, using Morris' predicted value for FVC in a 30-year-old man at a height of 71 inches, 1.1 L is subtracted from the predicted value of 5.56 L to obtain the 95 percent confidence lower limit of 4.46 L, which is 80 percent of the predicted value. For a 60-year-old man at a height of 63 inches, the same 1.1 L is subtracted from the value of 3.60 L to arrive at the 95 percent lower limit of 2.50 L, which is now 69 percent of the predicted value.

QUANTITATION OF ABNORMALITY

The *degree* of abnormality has generally been quantitated using percent of predicted value on a 4 or 5 point scale. Tables 9-1–9-6 show the categories of severity used. These scales have been based on clinical experience in correlating dyspnea with measured test results.

Should obstructive impairment be quantitated on the basis of FEV_1/FVC or FEV_1? Experience suggests that FEV_1/FVC is more useful for mild to moderate impairment and FEV_1 for advanced disease, when FVC is reduced by air trapping.

WHICH PREDICTION EQUATIONS TO USE?

Spirometry (FVC, FEV$_1$), Mean (FEF$_{25-75\%}$) and Instantaneous (FEF$_{50\%}$ and FEF$_{75\%}$) Maximum Flows (Tables 9-7 through 9-11)

It is increasingly recognized that well performed, reproducible spirometric tests may variously be interpreted as normal or abnormal depending on the choice of predicted values. Glindmeyer[13] pointed out an almost three-fold range of 140 to 360 cc per decade in the age coefficients for FVC and a range of 230 to 360 cc for FEV_1 in men. The FVC predicted for the same individual by the equations be analyzed varied by more than one liter (ca. 20 percent). The various equations are plotted in Figure 9-3 for VC or FVC, and Figure 9-4 for FEV_1.

In order to standardize the interpretation of spirometric tests, one set of predicted equations should be adopted. The Michigan equations are recommended because they are derived from a representative sample of the general population (in this case, of a large state). Instantaneous flows as well as spirometric measurements and SB D_LCO and TLC were analyzed. Variables are provided to account for the effect of cigarette smoking. The Michigan equations are similar to those of Crapo et al. from Utah[14] and Morris et al. from Oregon[15] when the difference in calculating FEV_1 is adjusted in the latter.

Single Breath Diffusing Capacity (Table 9-12)

The Michigan equations[2] are recommended for the following reasons. They are derived from a random sample of the general population. A large number of non-smokers and smokers were studied. They allow adjustment for the effect of cigarette smoking on D_LCO_{SB} in otherwise normal subjects. Use of D_LCO_{SB} values derived

Table 9-1

Quantitation of Impaired VC or FVC (Percent Predicted)

	Miller	Morris (1976)[25]	Sharpe (1979)[26]	Gaensler (1966)[27]	Ellis (1975)[28]	Morris (1984)[29]	Kanner (1975)[10]	Ostiguy (1979)[30]	Kanarek (personal communication)
Normal	≥80*	≥81	≥80	≥81	≥80	Within 1 CI	≥81	Within 2 SD	≥81
Slight (minimal)	70–79	65–80	70–79	60–80	64–79	1–1.75	66–80	61–normal	65–80
Moderate	55–69	50–64	55–69	50–59	44–63	1.75–2.5	51–65	40–60	50–64
Severe	40–50	35–49	45–54	35–49	<44	>2.5	≤50	<40	<49
Very Severe	<40	<35	<45	<35					

*We round off at the fourth decimal, eg. >79.5000; 79.4999 is not normal.

CI = Confidence interval, one-sided (1.645 SD)

SD = Standard deviation

Table 9-2
Quantitation of Impaired FEV$_1$ or MVV (Percent Predicted)

	Miller	Morris (1976)[25]	Snider (ACCP) (1967)[31]	Sharpe (1979)[26]	Gaensler* (1966)[27]	Ostiguy (1979)[30]	Kanarek (Personal communication)
Normal	≥80	≥81	≥80	≥80	≥81	Within 2 SD	≥81
Slight (minimal)	70–79	65–80	65–79	65–79	65–80	61–normal	60–80
Moderate	55–69	50–64	50–64	50–64	45–64	40–60	40–59
Severe	40–54	35–49	35–49	20–49	30–44	<40	≤39
Very Severe	<40	<35	<35	<20	<30		

*MVV only
SD = Standard Deviation

Table 9-3
Quantitation of Impaired MMF
($FEF_{25-75\%}$) (Percent Predicted)

	Miller	Morris* (1976)[25]	Ellis (1975)[28]
Normal	75–125	≥ 76	≥ 71
Slight (minimal)	60–74	60–75	
Moderate	40–59	45–59	
Severe	20–39	30–44	
Very Severe	< 20	< 30	

*Also $FEF_{200-1200}$, $FEF_{75-85\%}$.

only from nonsmokers will classify as impaired a large percentage of clinically normal smokers.

The lower values in current smokers and male exsmokers cannot be explained by back pressure of CO and may well indicate subclinical disease. The important point is that this impairment of gas exchange is attributable to the effects of cigarette smoking and must be distinguished from the effects of other disease processes or environmental exposures. Use of smoking-specific reference values permits this distinction to be made. Without smoking-specific values, it would be difficult to interpret a slightly or moderately decreased result in a patient with suspected ILD or a worker exposed to a pulmonary hazard who also smokes.

Findings using the newer Michigan equations are more or less comparable with those using the Gaensler equations,[16] which have been in wide use for more than a decade.

Maximum Voluntary Ventilation (Table 9-13)

Kory's values[17] for men and Lindall's[18] for women are recommended.

Total Lung Capacity, Functional Residual Capacity, and Residual Volume (Table 9-14)

The predicted values generated by the different equations vary markedly. As noted by Clausen[19], the value for RV of a 60-year-old male ranges from 1.84 to 2.83 L, for FRC from 2.76 to 4.06 L, and for TLC from 6.58 to 10.01 L.

Additionally, predicted values in use for measurements that are dependent each upon the other, such as RV, VC and TLC, have been derived from different series. One way to address this problem is to apply the VC/TLC (and therefore the RV/TLC) ratios reported by the references in this section to the VC standards utilized in your laboratory. In this way, consistent values for VC, TLC, and RV will be predicted.

Table 9-4

Quantitation of Impaired FEV_1/FVC

	Miller			Gaensler (1966)[27]	Ellis* (1975)[28]	Morris (1984)[29]	Kanner (1975)[10]	Kanarek (Personal communication)
	Age: ≤39	40–59	≥60					
Normal	0.75–0.89†	0.70–0.85†	0.65–0.85†	≥0.76	≥0.78	Within 1 CI	≥0.70	≥0.76
Slight (minimal)	0.65–0.74	0.60–0.69	0.60–0.64	0.60–0.75	0.67–0.77	1–2	0.61–0.69	0.60–0.75
Moderate	0.55–0.64	0.50–0.59	0.50–0.59	0.40–0.59	0.52–0.66	2–4	0.45–0.60	0.40–0.59
Severe	0.45–0.54	0.45–0.49	0.45–0.49	<0.40	<0.52	>4	<0.45	≤0.39
Very Severe	<0.45	<0.45	<0.45					

* After Cary (1979)[7] to convert from percent predicted.
† Values greater than these are considered high.
CI = confidence interval, one-sided (1.645 SD)

135

Table 9-5
Quantitation of Abnormal RV and TLC (Percent Predicted)

		Miller*	Gaensler RV (1966)[27]	Morris TLC or RV (1984)[29]	Kanner† (1975)[10]	
	RV	TLC			RV	TLC
Increase Very Severe	≥250		>200			>150
Severe	200–249		176–200	>2.0		135–149
Moderate	160–199	≥121	151–175	1.5–2.0	≥121	121–134
Slight	135–159		121–150	1.0–1.5		
Normal	80–134	80–120	80–120	Within 1 CI (TLC)	81–120	81–120
Decrease Slight	70–79			1.0–1.5		66–80
Moderate	60–69	≤79	<80	1.5–2.0	≤80	51–65
Severe	50–59			>2.0		≤50
Very Severe	<50					

*Plethysmography
†Single breath He dilution
CI = Confidence interval, two-sided (2 SD)

Table 9-6
Quantitation of Abnormal D_LCO_{SB} (Percent Predicted)

	Miller	Ellis (1975)[28]	Morris (1984)[29]	Kanner (1975)[10]	Kanarek (personal communication)	Ostiguy (1979)[30]
Normal	75–140*	≥80	Within 1 CI	81–140*		≥75
Slight (minimal)	65–74	64–79	1–1.75	61–80	≥71, exercise Δ(A-a) O_2 15–30 Torr	50–74
Moderate	50–64	44–63	1.75–2.5	41–60	40–70, exercise Δ(A-a) O_2 31–40 Torr	40–49
Severe	40–49	<44	>2.5	<41	≤39, exercise Δ(A-a) O_2 ≥ 41 Torr	<40
Very Severe	<40					

*Values greater than these are considered high.
CI = Confidence interval, one-sided (1.645 SD)

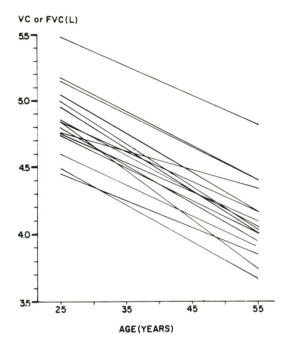

Fig. 9-3. Predicted VC or FVC for white males 68 inches in height, using various regression equations. [From Glindmeyer HW III. Predictable confusion. J. Occup Med 23:847, 1981, with permission.]

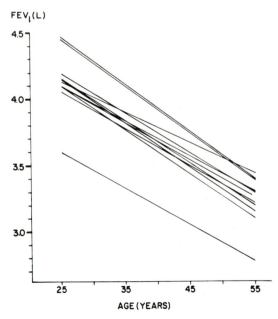

Fig. 9-4. Predicted FEV_1 for white males 68 inches in height, using various regression equations. [From Glindmeyer HW III. Predictable confusion. J Occup Med 23:847, 1981, with permission.]

Table 9-7

Prediction Equations for (Forced) Vital Capacity, White Adults (L)

Investigator	Smoking History	Intercept	Age	Height	R^2	SEE	95% Confidence Interval*
			Males				
Miller[1]	nonsmokers & current smokers	−7.750	−0.0212	+0.1965 in	0.57	0.510	0.838
Knudson[12]	nonsmokers	−8.782	−0.0298	+0.0844 cm	0.72	0.638	1.05
Crapo[14]	nonsmokers	−4.650	−0.0214	+0.0600 cm	0.54	0.644	1.115
Morris[15]	nonsmokers	−4.241	−0.025	+0.148 in	0.42	0.74	1.221
Kory[17]	mixed	−3.60	−0.022	+0.052 cm	0.64	0.58	0.96
			Females				
Miller[1]	nonsmokers & current smokers	−2.198	−0.0232	+0.1052 in	0.50	0.448	0.737
Knudson[12]	nonsmokers	−2.900	−0.0174	+0.0427 cm	0.54	0.493	0.81
Crapo[14]	nonsmokers	−3.590	−0.0216	+0.0491 cm	0.74	0.393	0.676
Morris[15]	nonsmokers	−2.852	−0.024	+0.115 in	0.50	0.52	0.858

*1.645 × SEE

Table 9-8
Prediction Equations for FEV_1, White Adults (L)

Investigator	Smoking History	Intercept	Age	Height	R^2	SEE	95% Confidence Interval*
			Males				
Miller[1]	nonsmokers	−4.908	−0.0233	+0.1438 in	0.61	0.412	0.68
Knudson[12]	nonsmokers	−6.515	−0.292	+0.067 cm	0.74	0.52	0.86
Crapo[14]	nonsmokers	−2.190	−0.0244	+0.0414 cm	0.64	0.486	0.84
Morris[15]	nonsmokers	−1.260	−0.032	+0.092 in	0.53	0.55	0.91
Kory[17]	mixed	−1.59	−0.028	+0.037 cm	0.63	0.52	0.86
			Females				
Miller[1]	nonsmokers & current smokers	−0.3801	−0.0251	+0.0681 in	0.61	0.332	0.55
Knudson[12]	nonsmokers	−1.405	−0.0201	+0.0309 cm	0.65	0.388	0.638
Crapo[14]	nonsmokers	−1.578	−0.0255	+0.0342 cm	0.80	0.326	0.56
Morris[15]	nonsmokers	−1.932	−0.025	+0.089 in	0.53	0.47	0.776

ND—No data.
*1.645 × SEE.

140

Table 9-9
Prediction Equations for MMF ($FEF_{25-75\%}$), White Adults (L/sec)

Investigator	Smoking History	Intercept	Age	Height	R^2	SEE	95% Confidence Interval*
			Males				
Miller[1]‡	nonsmokers	+0.301	−0.0096	+0.0206 in	0.31	0.234	0.385
Knudson[12]	nonsmokers	−4.518	−0.036	+0.058 cm	0.66	1.083	1.78
Crapo[14]	nonsmokers	+2.133	−0.0380	+0.0204 cm	0.42	0.962	1.666
Morris[15]	nonsmokers	+2.513	−0.045	+0.047 in	0.28	1.12	1.85
			Females				
Miller[1]‡	nonsmokers & current smokers	+1.563	−0.012	none	0.268	0.279	0.458
Knudson[12]	nonsmokers	+1.128	−0.034	+0.021 cm	0.67	0.842	1.38
Crapo[14]	nonsmokers	+2.683	−0.0460	+0.0154 cm	0.60	0.792	1.363
Morris[15]	nonsmokers	+0.551	−0.030	+0.06 in	0.31	0.80	1.32

*1.645 × SEE

‡Logarithm (natural); transform value to antilog

Table 9-10
Prediction Equations for $FEF_{50\%}$, White Adults (L/sec)

Investigator	Smoking History	No. of Subjects	Intercept	Age	Height	BSA (M²)	R²	SEE	95% Confidence Interval*
				Males					
Miller[1]‡	nonsmokers	190	+0.493	−0.0073	+0.0193 in	none	0.18	0.234	0.38
Knudson[12]	nonsmokers	86	−5.541	−0.037	+0.068 cm	none	0.38	1.29	2.13
Black[22]	mixed	83	+7.374	−0.052	none	none	ND	1.29	2.13
Bass[32]	nonsmokers	149	+9.45	−0.038	−0.107 in	+2.35	0.38	1.34	2.21
Cherniack[33]	nonsmokers	870	+2.403	−0.030	+0.065 in	none	0.27	ND	ND
				Females					
Miller[1]‡	nonsmokers & current smokers	206	+1.636	−0.0082	none	none	0.16	0.265	0.44
Knudson[12]	nonsmokers	204	+0.609	−0.029	+0.027 cm	none	0.33	0.971	1.60
Black[22]	mixed	110	+4.978	−0.025	none	none	ND	1.09	1.79
Bass[32]	nonsmokers	98	+5.37	−0.029	none	none	0.37	1.1	1.82
Cherniack[33]	nonsmokers	452	+1.426	−0.023	+0.062 in	none	0.36	ND	ND

ND—No data
*1.645 × SEE
‡Logarithm (natural); transform value to antilog

Table 9-11
Prediction Equations for $FEF_{75\%}$, White Adults (L/sec)

Investigator	Smoking History	No. of Subjects	Intercept	Age	Height	BSA (M²)	R²	SEE	95% Confidence Interval*
				Males					
Miller[1]‡	nonsmokers	190	−0.540	−0.0186	+0.0267 in	none	0.49	0.282	0.46
Knudson[12]	nonsmokers	86	−2.483	−0.023	+0.031 cm	none	0.40	0.692	1.13
Black[22]	mixed	83	+3.673	−0.042	none	none	ND	0.60	0.99
Bass[32]	nonsmokers	149	+1.61	−0.024	none	+0.613	0.42	0.71	1.17
Cherniack[33]	nonsmokers	870	+1.984	−0.041	+0.036 in	none	0.62	ND	ND
				Females					
Miller[1]‡	nonsmokers & current	206	+1.112	−0.0197	none	none	0.35	0.374	0.62
Knudson[12]	nonsmokers	204	+1.118	−0.026	+0.010 cm	none	0.42	0.65	1.07
Black[22]	mixed	110	+2.469	−0.025	none	none	ND	0.49	0.81
Bass[32]	nonsmokers	98	+2.59	−0.023	none	none	0.5	0.58	0.96
Cherniack[33]	nonsmokers	452	+2.216	−0.034	+0.023 in	none	0.44	ND	ND

ND—No data
*1.645 × SEE
‡Logarithm (natural); transform value to antilog

Table 9-12
Prediction Equations for D_LCO_{SB}, Adults, ml/Torr/min

SMOKING NOT TAKEN INTO ACCOUNT

Gaensler[16]	98 normal subjects; ≥ 50% smokers	M = 0.250 Ht (in) − 0.177 Age + 19.93 F = 0.284 Ht (in) − 0.177 Age + 7.72
Cotes[34]	ND	M = 2.99* × [10.9 Ht (m) − 0.067 Age − 5.89]

SMOKING TAKEN INTO ACCOUNT

Van Ganse[35]	142; 53 nonsmokers (16 men)	M = 16.36 Ht (m) − 0.202 Age − 0.42 LP + 9.711 (±3.82) F = 16.80 Ht (m) − 0.157 Age − 0.21 LP + 0.339 (±3.59) LP = lifetime packs/1000
Crapo[36]	245 normal nonsmokers	M (nonsmoker) = 0.416 Ht (cm) − 0.219 Age − 26.34 (±4.82) F (nonsmoker) = 0.256 Ht (cm) − 0.144 Age − 8.36 (±3.60)
Miller[2]	511 subjects; 204 nonsmokers, 218 smokers, 89 ex-smokers; random selection of State of Michigan	M (nonsmoker) = 0.418 Ht (in) − 0.229 Age − 12.9113 (±4.84) M (smoker) = 0.418 Ht (in) − 0.229 Age + 7.5195 (±4.84) M (exsmoker) = 0.418 Ht (in) − 0.229 Age − 10.6546 (±4.84) F (nonsmoker)† = 0.407 Ht (in) − 0.111 Age − 2.2382 (±3.95) F (smoker) = 0.407 Ht (in) − 0.111 Age − 1.3227 (±3.95)

ND—No data
*Converts SIU to traditional units; 0.334 converts traditional units to SIU
†Includes exsmokers

Table 9-13

Prediction Equations for MVV, White Adults (L/min)

Investigator	No. of Subjects	Intercept	Age	Height	BSA (M²)	R²	SEE	95% Confidence Interval*
				Males				
Bass[32]	149	−76.8	−0.814	+3.65 in	none	0.48	25.2	41.6
Kory[17]	464	−21.4	−1.26	+1.34 cm	none	0.29	29.0	47.9
Needham[37]†	102	+94	−1.1	none	+40	ND	18	29.7
Baldwin[38]	52	(+86.5	−0.522)	none	×1.0	ND	ND	ND
				Females				
Bass[32]	98	127.4	−0.692	none	none	0.53	16.5	27.2
Lindall[18]	101	−5.5	−0.57	+2.05 in	none	ND	15.4	25.3
Needham[37]†	66	+113	−0.7	none	none	ND	13	21.4
Baldwin[38]	40	(+71.3	−0.474)	none	×1.0	ND	ND	ND

ND—No Data

*1.645 × SEE

†values ATPS

145

Table 9-14

Prediction Equations for TLC, FRC, and RV, White Adults (L)

Investigator	No. of Subjects	Lung Volume	Method	Intercept	Age	Height	BSA (M²)	Weight	R²	SEE	95% Confidence Interval*
Males											
O'Brien[39]	416	TLC	R	−12.43	+0.01	+0.013 cm	−2.36	None	0.47	0.74	1.21
	329	RV		−2.60	+0.03	+0.002 cm	None	+0.01 kg	0.40	0.56	0.93
Black[22]	83	TLC	P(V)	−6.806	None	+0.078 cm	None	None	0.60	0.68	1.12
		RV		−6.026	+0.034	+0.038 cm	None	None	0.61	0.57	0.94
Boren[21]	422	TLC	MB	−7.30	None	+0.078 cm	None	None	0.56	0.87	1.43
		FRC		−2.94	None	+0.032 cm	None	None	0.36	0.63	1.04
		RV		−2.24	+0.0115	+0.019 cm	None	None	0.33	0.53	0.87
Goldman[20]†	44	TLC	MB	−9.167	−0.015	+0.094 cm	None	None	0.77	ND	ND
		FRC		−7.11	None	+0.081 cm	−1.79	None	0.57	ND	ND
		RV		−3.447	+0.017	+0.027 cm	None	None	0.64	ND	ND
Females											
O'Brien[39]	1393	TLC	R	−7.62	+0.01	+0.008 cm	None	−0.01 kg	0.41	0.56	0.93
	926	RV		−4.78	+0.03	+0.004 cm	−0.73	None	0.44	0.49	0.80
Black[22]	110	TLC	P(V)	−5.359	None	+0.064 cm	None	None	0.53	0.62	1.02
		RV		−2.978	+0.021	+0.023 cm	None	None	0.49	0.46	0.76
Goldman[20]†	50	TLC	MB	−7.49	−0.008	+0.079 cm	None	None	0.72	ND	ND
		FRC		−4.74	None	+0.53 cm	None	+0.017 kg	0.61	ND	ND
		RV		−3.90	+0.009	+0.032 cm	None	None	0.55	ND	ND

*1.654 × SEE
†Values ATPS
ND = No data; R = Radiographic; P(V) = Plethysomography (volume displacement); MB = Multiple breath.

Table 9-15
Prediction Equations for PFR, White Adults (L/sec)

Investigator	No. of Subjects	Instrument	Intercept	Age	Height	BSA (M²)	R²	SEE	95% Confidence Interval*
				Males					
Montner[40]	54	rolling seal spirometer	+4.60	−0.03	+0.23 in	ND	0.21	ND	ND
Knudson[41]	128	pneumotach	−5.993	−0.035	+0.094 cm	ND	0.24	2.078	3.43
Higgins[42]	1035	wedge spirometer	−1.616	−0.036	+0.065 cm	ND	0.35	1.858	3.07
Bass[32]	149	wedge spirometer	+4.63	−0.026	None	+2.38	0.31	1.48	2.44
Cherniack[33]	870	wedge spirometer	+0.225	−0.024	+0.144 in	ND	0.27	ND	ND
Leiner[43]§	105	PF meter	(+3.95)	−0.0151)	×1 cm	None	ND	ND	ND
				Females					
Montner[40]	68	rolling seal spirometer	+3.16	−0.04	+0.09 in	ND	0.39	ND	ND
Knudson[41]	321	pneumotach	−0.735	−0.025	+0.049 cm	ND	0.15	1.605	2.64
Higgins[42]	1285	wedge spirometer	+0.726	+0.020	+0.034 cm	ND	0.25	1.321	2.18
Bass[32]	98	wedge spirometer	+2.72	−0.028 (Weight,	None −0.017 lbs)	+3.93	0.43	1.13	1.86
Cherniack[33]	452	wedge spirometer	+1.131	−0.178	0.091 in	ND	0.26	ND	ND
Leiner[43]§	50	PF meter	(+2.93)	−0.0072)	×1 cm	None	ND	ND	ND

*1.645 × SEE
§L/min

147

Although Goldman's (1959) values[20] are widely used, they were derived from a small number of subjects at high altitude. Boren's (1966)[21] are unfortunately available only for males. We have used Black's (1974),[22] since they were based on 193 subjects and utilized a plethysmographic method; values are not given for FRC.

Peak Flow Rate (Table 9-15)

Maximum Respiratory Pressures

The most widely used reference is Black and Hyatt.[23,24]

References

1. Miller A, Thornton JC, Warshaw R, et al. Mean and instantaneous expiratory flows, FVC and FEV_1: Prediction equations from a probability sample of Michigan, a large industrial state. Bull Physiopath Resp, in press.
2. Miller A, Thornton JC, Warshaw R, et al. Single breath diffusing capacity in a representative sample of the population of Michigan, a large industrial state: Predicted values, lower limits of normal, and frequencies of abnormality by smoking history. Am Rev Respir Dis 127:270–277, 1983
3. Fletcher CM. Terminology in chronic obstructive lung disease. J. Epidemiol Comm Health 32:282–288, 1978
4. Rossiter CE, Weill H. Ethnic differences in lung function. Evidence for proportional differences. Int J Epidemiol 3:55–61, 1974
5. Miller WF, Johnson RL Jr, Wu N. Relationship between fast vital capacity and various timed expiratory capacities. J Appl Physiol 14:157–163, 1959
6. Stuart DG, Collings WD. Comparison of vital capacity and maximum breathing capacity of athletes and non-athletes. J Appl Physiol 14:507–509, 1959
7. Shapiro W, Patterson JF Jr. Effects of smoking and athletic conditioning on ventilatory mechanics including observations on the reliability of the forced expirogram. Am Rev Respir Dis 85:191–199, 1962
8. Crosbie WA, Clarke MB, Cox RAF, et al. Physical characteristics and ventilatory function of 404 commercial divers working in the North Sea. Br J Ind Med 34:19–25, 1977
9. Wilson K, Miller W, Blair T, et al. Flow-volume relationships in obstructive and restrictive lung disease. Chest 70:445, 1976
10. Kanner RE, Morris AH (Eds). Clinical pulmonary function testing. A manual of uniform laboratory procedures for the intermountain area. Salt Lake City, Intermountain Thoracic Society, 1975
11. Kuperman AS, Riker JB. The predicted normal maximal midexpiratory flow rate. AM Rev Respir Dis 107:231–238, 1973
12. Knudson RJ, Lebowitz MD, Holberg CJ, et al. Changes in the normal maximal expiratory flow-volume curve with growth and aging. Am Rev Respir Dis 127:725–734, 1983
13. Glindmeyer HW III. Predictable confusion. J Occup Med 23:845–849, 1981

14. Crapo RO, Morris AH, Gardner RM. Reference spirometric values using techniques and equipment that meet ATS recommendations. Am Rev Respir Dis 123:659–644, 1981

15. Morris JF, Koski A, Johnson LC. Spirometric standards for healthy nonsmoking adults. Am Rev Respir Dis 103:57–67, 1971

16. Gaensler EA, Smith AA. Attachment for automated single breath diffusing capacity measurement. Chest 63:136–145, 1973

17. Kory RC, Callahan R, Boren HG, et al. The Veterans Administration–Army cooperative study of pulmonary function. I. Clinical spirometry in normal men. Am J Med 30:243–258, 1961

18. Lindall A, Medina A, Grismer JT. A re-evaluation of normal pulmonary function measurements in the adult female. Am Rev Respir Dis 95:1061–1064, 1967

19. Clausen JL (Ed). Pulmonary function testing. Guidelines and controversies. Equipment, methods, and normal values. New York, Academic Press, 1982

20. Goldman HI, Becklake MR. Respiratory function tests. Normal values at median altitudes and the prediction of normal results. Am Rev Respir Dis 79:457–467, 1959

21. Boren HG, Kory RC, Syner JC. The Veterans Administration–Army cooperative study of pulmonary function. II. The lung volume and its subdivisions in normal men. Am J Med 41:96–114, 1966

22. Black LF, Offord K, Hyatt RE. Variability in the maximal expiratory flow volume curve in asymptomatic smokers and nonsmokers. Am Rev Respir Dis 110:282–292, 1974

23. Black LF, Hyatt RE. Maximal respiratory pressures: Normal values and relationship to age and sex. Am Rev Respir Dis 99:696–702, 1969

24. Black LF, Hyatt RE. Maximal static respiratory pressures in generalized neuromuscular disease. Am Rev Respir Dis 103:641–650, 1971

25. Morris JF. Spirometry in the evaluation of pulmonary function. West J Med 125:110–118, 1976

26. Sharpe IK, Tomashefsky JF. The physician's role in the evaluation of disability due to pulmonary disease. Clin Notes Resp Dis 17:3–12, 1979

27. Gaensler EA, Wright GW. Evaluation of respiratory impairment. Arch Environ Health 12:146–189, 1966

28. Ellis JH Jr, Perera SP, Levin DC. A computer program for calculation and interpretation of pulmonary function studies. Chest 68:209–213, 1975

29. Morris AH, Kanner RE, Crapo RO, et al. Clincial pulmonary function testing: A Manual of Uniform Laboratory Procedures (ed 2). Salt Lake City, Intermountain Thoracic Society, 1984

30. Ostiguy GL. Summary of task force report on occupational respiratory disease (pneumonconiosis). Can Med Ass J 121:414–421, 1979

31. Snider GL, Kory RC, Lyons HA. Grading of pulmonary function impairment by means of pulmonary function tests. Recommendations of the Commitee on Pulmonary Physiology, American College of Chest Physicians. Dis Chest 52:270–271, 1967

32. Bass H. The flow volume loop: Normal standards and abnormalities in chronic obstructive pulmonary disease. Chest 63:171–176, 1973

33. Cherniack RM, Raber MB. Normal standards for ventilatory function using an automated wedge spirometer. Am Rev Respir Dis 106:38–46, 1972

34. Cotes JE. Lung function (4th ed). Oxford, Blackwell Scientific, 1979

35. Van Ganse WF, Ferris BG Jr, Cotes JE. Cigarette smoking and pulmonary diffusing capacity (Transfer factor). Am Rev Respir Dis 105:30–41, 1972

36. Crapo RO, Morris AH. Standardized single breath normal values for carbon monoxide diffusing capacity. Am Rev Respir Dis 123:185–189, 1981

37. Needham CD, Rogan MC, McDonald I. Normal standards for lung volumes, intrapulmonary gas mixing, and maximum breathing capacity. Thorax 9:313–325, 1954

38. Baldwin EF, Cournand A, Richards DW. Pulmonary insufficiency. I. Physiological classification, clinical methods of analysis, standard values in normal subjects. Medicine 27:243–278, 1948

39. O'Brien RD, Drizd TA. Roentgenographic determination of total lung capacity: Normal values from a national population survey. Am Rev Respir Dis 128:949–952, 1983

40. Montner P, Miller A, Calhoun F. Tracheal diameter as a predictor of pulmonary function. Lung 162:115–121, 1984

41. Knudson RJ, Slatin RC, Lebowitz MD, et al. The maximal expiratory flow–volume curve. Normal standards, variability and effects of age. Am Rev Resp Dis 113:587–600, 1976

42. Higgins MW, Keller JB. Seven measures of ventilatory lung function. Population values and a comparison of their study to discriminate between persons with and without chronic respiratory symptoms and disease, Tecumseh, Michigan. Am Rev Respir Dis 108:258–272, 1973

43. Leiner GC, Abramowitz S, Small MJ, et al. Expiratory peak flow rate: Standard values for normal subjects. Use as a clinical test of ventilatory function. Am Rev Respir Dis 88:644–651, 1963

10

Patterns of Impairment

Albert Miller

Obstructive Impairment (Airways Obstruction or Airflow Limitation)
　Upper versus Lower Airways
　　Upper
　　Lower
　Large (Central) versus Small (Peripheral) Airways
　　Flow Characteristics
　Small Airways Obstruction
　　Recognition
　　The Spectrum of Small Airways Obstruction
　Overt Airways Obstruction
　　Characteristic Findings
　　Distinguishing Emphysema From Obstructive Bronchitis and Asthma
　　Dynamic Airway Collapse
　　Bullous Disease
　　Endogenous Factors in CAO
　　Other Causes of Overt Airways Obstruction
　Reversibility
Restrictive Impairment
　Definition
　　Total Lung Capacity Decreased
　　Total Lung Capacity and Residual Volume "Not Increased"
　The Limitation in using the Vital Capacity to Define Restriction
　　Clues to Air Trapping When the FVC is Reduced

PULMONARY FUNCTION TESTS: A　　ISBN 0-8089-1764-4　Copyright © 1987 by Grune & Stratton
GUIDE FOR THE STUDENT AND HOUSE OFFICER　　All rights of reproduction in any form reserved.

Types of Restriction
  Diffuse Pulmonary Disease
  Resection and Autopneumonectomy
  Chest Wall (or Chest Bellows) Disorders:
    Skeletal Deformities
    Pleural Disease
    Increased Abdominal Pressure, Obesity
    Reduced Force Generation, Neuromuscular Disease
Combined (Restrictive-Obstructive) Impairment
  Combined Impairment Due to a Single Disease Process
    Chronic Granulomatous Disease
    Cystic Fibrosis and Bronchiectasis
    Silicosis and Coal Workers' Pneumoconiosis
    Congestive Heart Failure
  Airways Function in Interstitital Lung Disease
    Small Airways Obstruction
    Overt Airways Obstruction
  Superimposition of Disease Processes
Isolated Diffusion Defect
  Interstitial Lung Disease
  Pulmonary Vascular Disease
  Anemia and Abnormal Hemoglobin,
Respiratory Center Unresponsiveness
Abnormal Blood Gases in the Absence of Other Pulmonary
  Function Abnormalities
  Hypoxemia
    Chest Bellows Disorders
    Small Airways Obstruction
    ILD
    Venoarterial Shunt
  Hypercapnia

The results of pulmonary function tests seldom *establish the clinical diagnosis;* they do form patterns of impairment that *suggest, confirm* or *help rule out* various disease states.

OBSTRUCTIVE IMPAIRMENT (AIRWAYS OBSTRUCTION OR AIRFLOW LIMITATION)

Upper Versus Lower Airways

Upper

Upper airways obstruction is discussed in detail and illustrated in Chapter 3.

Lower

By far the greatest number of patients with objective respiratory difficulties have lower airways obstruction. If not otherwise specified, "obstructive airways disease" or any synonymous term refers to the lower airways.

Large (Central) versus Small (Peripheral) Airways

Flow Characteristics

Flow in the large airways.   Large airways are those with diameters greater than 2 mm and they include the first 9 generations. Weibel[1] and Horsfield and Cumming[2] made precise measurements of the number of branches and their diameters and calculated total cross-sectional area and resistance to airflow at different levels in the tracheobronchial tree. They noted relatively little change in cross-sectional area until the 9th generation. The greatest pressure drop during airflow took place from the 5th to 9th generations, where the increased resistance in the smaller daughter bronchi was not accompanied by an increase in their cross-sectional area. Macklem and Mead,[3] using a retrograde catheter, estimated that about 75 percent of the total pressure drop occurred in these central airways.

Flow in the small airways (See Chapter 6).   Beyond the 9th generation, total cross-sectional area increases rapidly. The greatest increase takes place at the terminal and first generation of respiratory bronchioles. According to prevailing opinion, since less than 25 percent of total resistance to airflow is in these peripheral airways, a large increase in their resistance would not affect overall airway resistance as measured clinically. The G_{aw}, FEV_1, FEV_1/FVC, PFR, and MVV would accordingly not be reduced.

Recently, certain investigators[4,5] have increased the contributions of the peripheral airways to total resistance and concepts of small airways disease may be changing.

Small Airways Obstruction

Recognition

From the spirogram and MEFV curve, small airways (SA) obstruction is recognized by reduced flows at low lung volumes ($FEF_{25-75\%}$, $FEF_{75-85\%}$, $FEF_{50\%}$, $FEF_{75\%}$) while FVC and FEV_1 are normal.

In patients with SA obstruction, the RV and RV/TLC are often increased, as are the SB N_2 difference and/or closing volume (or closing capacity). In the presence of normal R_{aw} and static lung compliance, lung compliance is frequency-dependent at respiratory rates $\geq 60/min$; ie, compliance falls ≥ 25 percent. Dynamic compliance at the resting respiratory rate is similar to static compliance, unlike the findings in emphysema. (Frequency dependence of compliance and washout tests are even more abnormal in overt airways obstruction than in SA obstruction, but R_{aw} and/or static compliance are also abnormal.

As a practical matter, many individuals are encountered who demonstrate one or more of the following: decreased flows at low lung volumes, increased RV, increased SB N_2 gradient and/or closing volume, abnormal response to hel-ox, and frequency dependence of compliance in the presence of normal FVC, FEV_1, FEV_1/FVC, static compliance, and R_{aw}. Most of these individuals fall into certain categories: cigarette smokers, asthmatics in remission, patients with early left ventricular failure (eg, having had acute myocardial infarction), patients with recent respiratory infection, and those with exposure to noxious fumes.

The Spectrum of Small Airways Obstruction

The term "small airways obstruction" has been applied to two very different clinical situations.

"Minimal airways dysfunction." This is what is usually meant by "small airways obstruction." Used as a *physiologic* description, it is accompanied *anatomically* by obstructive changes in the peripheral airways that are evidence of damage from cigarette smoke and other noxious (including infectious) inhalants. Clinical and radiographic examination and "routine" pulmonary function tests are changed minimally or not at all. Thus the pathologic alterations are in the "silent zones" of the lungs. They are detectable by the various physiologic tests outlined above.

From the pathologic changes in the peripheral airways, other physiologic abnormalities ensue, such as ventilation-perfusion imbalance, increased alveolar-arterial difference in PO_2, increased dead space, and slight to moderate hypoxemia. These abnormalities do not cause symptoms, let alone respiratory insufficiency. They are present in many individuals who are not only asymptomatic but who remain asymptomatic for many years or for the remainder of their lives. (Since up to 50 percent of smokers exhibit physiologic and presumably anatomic evidence of small airways obstruction yet only about 10 percent eventuate in CAO, it may be inferred that in most smokers, small airways obstruction does not portend progressive obstructive airways disease.)

Many thoughtful physicians consider the finding of minimal airways dysfunction to be without *immediate* clinical importance. If the patient presents with dyspnea, it should not be attributed to this finding.

The small airways in chronic airways obstruction. The other meaning of the term small airways disease has also been in use for more than a decade. It refers to the major site of pathologic alteration in patients who have clinical and physiologic findings typical of CAO and whose pulmonary function tests show overt airways obstruction.

Thus, when a patient manifests overt airways obstruction, anatomic changes may be predominantly in the small airways. Elastic recoil may be normal, as in the cases described by Macklem, Thurlbeck, and Fraser,[6] who showed very little emphysema; or decreased, as in the patients with obvious anatomic emphysema described by Hogg, Macklem and Thurlbeck[7] in 1968.

Overt Airways Obstruction

Characteristic Findings

This term refers to the typical functional changes seen in acute or chronic asthma, obstructive bronchitis and emphysema. The FEV_1 and FEV_1/FVC are decreased. Airway resistance is increased; specific airway conductance (SG_{aw}) is decreased. Peak flow is decreased and flow rates at mid and low lung volume ($FEF_{25-75\%}$, $FEF_{50\%}$, $FEF_{75\%}$) are markedly decreased.

The RV and to a lesser degree, the TLC, are increased. The VC and FVC may be normal but are decreased in more severe disease; the slow VC is often larger than the FVC.

The MVV is decreased proportionally to the degree of obstruction. The observed MVV usually approximates the value predicted from the FEV_1 unless respiratory muscle fatigue is present. The air velocity index or percent predicted MVV/percent predicted VC is < 1.0.

Distinguishing Emphysema from Obstructive Bronchitis and Asthma

Emphysema cannot be separated from the other causes of CAO by indices of airflow or by any of the tests outlined above. Emphysema means destruction of lung parenchyma, including elastic tissue and capillary bed. This is reflected in a decreased elastic recoil (or increased static compliance) and a decreased D_L (and D_L/V_A). These tests can be used to distinguish emphysema from chronic bronchitis or asthma.

Destruction of elastic tissue and decreased recoil of the lung result in a generally larger RV and TLC in patients with emphysema but the values for these measurements overlap the values seen in obstructive bronchitis and asthma.

Dynamic Airway Collapse

This subject is also discussed in Chapter 2 and illustrated in Figure 10-1. Dynamic compression occurs to some extent in normal airways during forced expiration, as may be observed with the fiberoptic bronchoscope. When elastic support of the large airways is lost in emphysema, dynamic compression is far greater and may cause brief total collapse. This is associated with a characteristic pattern of the MEVF curve showing the following.[8]

1. An abrupt decrease in flow from a well-defined (although reduced) peak.
2. The inflection point is reached within the first 25 percent of the FVC.
3. The remainder of the FVC is delivered at a more-or-less unvarying low flow rate, often ≤ 0.2 L/sec.

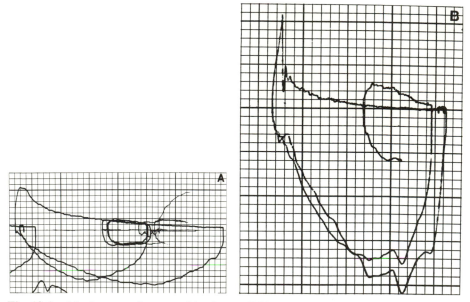

Fig. 10-1. Maximum expiratory and inspiratory F-V curves showing the pattern of dynamic collapse. (A) FVC only slightly reduced (3.63 L, 74 percent of predicted). The patient is a 38-year-old male exsmoker with alpha-1 antiprotease deficiency (Case Presentation 10-1). (B) FVC markedly reduced secondary to air trapping (1.92 L, 39 percent of predicted). The patient is a 38-year-old male exsmoker with normal alpha-1 antiprotease levels but other findings very similar to (A): FEV_1 0.57 L (16 percent of predicted), RV 6.21 L (303 percent of predicted). TLC 8.52 L (127 percent of predicted). Volume 1 L per large division, flow 2 L/sec per large division.

The FVC itself may or may not be very reduced (Fig. 10-1 A and B, respectively). A MEFV curve showing dynamic collapse is typical but not pathognomonic of emphysema, since it may be seen in bronchiolitis obliterans (see below).

The patient must generate sufficient intrapleural pressure to demonstrate a curve showing dynamic collapse. With less effort (<40 percent of maximal intrapleural pressure), the typical contour is not seen and flows at mid and low lung volumes are higher. Thus, tidal flows exceed "maximal" flows.

Bullous Disease

Bullae in otherwise normal lungs. Bullae (thin-walled, often multiloculated, air-filled spaces) may be seen in otherwise normal lungs. On pulmonary function testing, their presence is suggested by an increase in RV measured plethysmographically, with a large difference between plethysmographic and dilutional lung volumes, which represents the "trapped gas" within the bullae. Because the air-filled spaces compress normal lung, the spirometric pattern may be "restrictive." Indeed, this is a fair characterization of the impairment when the lungs are otherwise normal. The R_{aw} is often not elevated and the FEV_1/FVC and flows derived from the spirogram and MEFV curve may be normal or high.

Bullae in generalized emphysema. More commonly, bullae are part of generalized emphysema. Physiologic evidence of airflow limitation and emphysema is then present, as is apparent from the pulmonary function tests shown in Table 10-1. Note the striking 5.0 L decrease in RV, 2.2 L increase in FVC, and 750 cc increase in FEV_1 following surgical removal of the bullae in the left upper lobe. The bullae as they were seen at surgery are shown in Figure 10-2, along with the initial chest roentgenographs.

Endogenous Factors in CAO

Alpha1-antiprotease deficiency. The association between CAO and a deficiency in antiprotease activity was first noted in 1963 by Laurell and Eriksson.[9] Most patients with severe (homozygous) deficiency manifest symptomatic CAO by age 40 years in the absence of chronic bronchitis.[10] Pulmonary function findings are characteristic of emphysema. Radiographic changes (avascularity and bullae) are

Table 10-1
Pulmonary Function Before and Three Months
After Resection of a Bulla in a 69-Year-Old
White Male Smoker, 165 cm, 71 kg*

	6/80	10/80
Lung Volumes		
VC (cc)	1750 (45%)	3660 (100%)
ERV	700	1120
FRC (plet)	9050	4460
TLC	10100 (157%)	7000 (112%)
RV	8350 (312%)	3340 (128%)
Spirometry and Flows		
FVC (cc)	1480 (41%)	3660 (100%)
FEV_1	510 (21%)	1260 (51%)
FEV_1/FVC	0.34	0.35
FEV_3/FVC	—	0.65
PFR (L/sec)	—	3.87
$FEF_{25-75\%}$	0.16 (7%)	0.52 (21%)
MVV (L/min)	—	61 (69%)
D_LCO_{SB} (cc/min/Torr)	—	10.8 (58%)†
D_LCO/TLC_{SB}	—	1.96 (57%)†

†Predicted value for current smokers; D_LCO_{SB} is 44 percent and D_LCO/TLC_{SB} 46 percent of values for nonsmokers.
*See footnote to Table 1-1, page 7, for description of predicted values used for tables showing pulmonary function results.

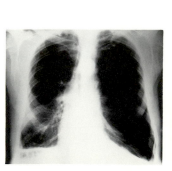
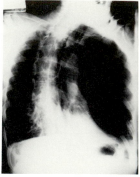
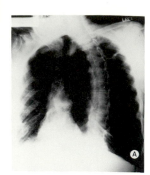

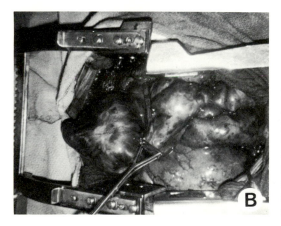

Fig. 10-2. (A) Chest radiographs in posteroanterior and both oblique projections showing bullae in both upper lobes compressing the lower zones. The left-sided bulla occupies at least 80 percent of the hemithorax and has displaced the mediastinum and heart to the right. (B) Appearance of the bullae at thoracotomy.

more prominent at the bases in contrast to more marked upper zone abnormalities in other patients with emphysema, as illustrated in Case Presentation 10-1.

This is a 38-year old-Hispanic male who had smoked two packages of cigarettes a day from age 15 years through age 36 years. He presented with progressive dyspnea of two years' duration and productive cough. On physical examination, the chest was hyperresonant, breath sounds were decreased and expiration prolonged. Right atrial hypertrophy was present on the electrocardiogram. On pulmonary function testing (Table 10-2), severe airways obstruction, hyperinflation, and diminution in D_LCO_{SB} were apparent. His MEFV curve demonstrating dynamic airway collapse is seen in Figure 10-1A. Because he was young for such emphysema and because of the basal bullae seen on chest radiograph (Fig. 10-3), a serum alpha$_1$-antiprotease level was obtained and found to be markedly reduced (30 mg/100 cc, normal 200–400). Liver biopsy showed D-PAS globules containing alpha$_1$-antiprotease in the cytoplasm of the hepatocytes.

Hypocomplementemic urticarial vasculitis. This disorder provides another illustration of the interaction of endogenous and environmental factors in CAO.

Table 10-2
Case Presentation 10-1, Emphysema
Due to Alpha-1 Antiprotease
Deficiency in a 38-year-old Hispanic
Male Exsmoker, 173 cm, 53 kg

	1/83
Lung Volumes	
VC (cc)	3240 (66%)
ERV	700
FRC (plet)	5940
TLC	8480 (121%)
RV	5240 (241%)
Spirometry and Flows	
FVC (cc)	3240 (66%)
FEV_1	980 (26%)
FEV_1/FVC	0.30
FEV_3/FVC	0.57
PFR (L/sec)	2.5
$FEF_{25-75\%}$	0.36 (9%)
MVV (L/min)	28 (26%)
D_LCO_{SB} (cc/min/Torr)	10.4 (35%)
D_LCO/TLC_{SB}	2.16 (46%)
PaO_2, rest, Torr	72
PaO_2, exercise	39

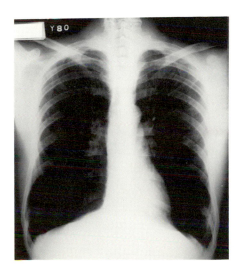 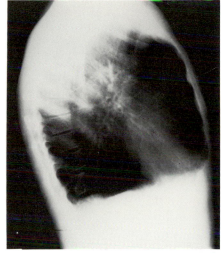

Fig. 10-3. (Case Presentation 10-1) PA and lateral chest radiographs showing emphysema in a 38-year-old exsmoker with alpha-1 antiprotease deficiency. In addition to the flattened diaphragm and increase in anteroposterior diameter and retrosternal air space, note the greater radiolucency at both bases. Bullous change in the lower zones is characteristic of emphysema due to antiprotease deficiency.

During a 14-year follow-up of 10 smokers with this immunologic disorder, eight developed CAO at an early age.[11]

Other Causes of Overt Airways Obstruction

Bronchiolitis obliterans. Turton[12] reviewed 2094 consecutive patients with overt airways obstruction and excluded those with a history or evidence of smoking, asthma, chronic bronchitis, emphysema, congestive heart failure, or specific pulmonary disease. Ten patients remained who were thought to have bronchiolitis obliterans. The diagnosis was confirmed by bronchography in three patients. Physiologically, patients showed increased R_{aw}, decreased FVC, FEV_1/FVC, and flows, and air trapping. The MEFV curves demonstrated dynamic collapse, although compliance was normal, as was D_L/V_A. The authors hypothesized that the reduction in FVC reflected the degree of closure of small airways. The course of the disease was slow.

Seggev et al[13] reported histologic findings in three cases of bronchiolitis obliterans. These consisted of obliteration and narrowing of small bronchioles, with polypoid masses of granulation tissue obstructing the lumina.

Bronchiolitis obliterans is often associated with organizing pneumonia. Epler[14] described polypoid granulation tissue and fibrosis in the lumens of small airways, alveolar ducts, and alveoli. The clinical presentation (often following a flu-like illness), and radiographic changes (patchy densities) were consistent with an organizing pneumonia. The physiologic findings of restriction and decreased D_L differentiated this disorder from "bronchiolitis obliterans with irreversible obstruction" described above. The uniform age of the pathologic reaction, the response to corticosteroids and the favorable prognosis distinguished the syndrome from "usual interstitial pneumonitis." Causes of bronchiolitis obliterans include toxic fume inhalation (NO_2, Cl_2), or virus, *Mycoplasma,* or *Pertussis* infection, especially in children. Vasculitis is also a cause; of Turton's ten cases, five had underlying rheumatoid arthritis. Bronchiolitis obliterans has been reported after penicillamine therapy of this disease.[15]

Chronic graft versus host disease is also a cause. Severe CAO with bronchiolitis obliterans on lung biopsy has been increasingly reported in this setting in previously well young nonsmokers. Onset may be isidious, 9–22 months after allogeneic bone marow transplantation.[16] The disorder may stabilize or result in death from obstructive respiratory failure.[17]

Comment. Bronchiolitis obliterans is emerging as a cause of CAO. It can be mistaken for interstitial fibrosis and organizing pneumonia at one extreme and for emphysema at the other. Functional findings which are central to the diagnosis of bronchiolitis obliterans causing CAO are irreversibility, air trapping (without the tremendous increase in RV and TLC characteristic of emphysema) and perhaps, preserved DL/VA. It is undoubtedly more common than reports indicate since it may be present in smokers, who are then diagnosed as chronic bronchitis and/or emphysema; patients with some reversibility on inhalation of a BD, who are then diagnosed as asthma; and patients who have ILD and airways obstruction (see section below).

Ciliary dyskinesia (immotile cilia syndrome).   The impairment of ciliary clearance is caused by various ultrastructural defects in respiratory cilia. It is often associated with irreversible obstructive impairment and air trapping as well as bronchiectasis and chronic rhinitis, otitis, and sinusitis.

Reversibility

Reversibility is established by an increase in flow (conventionally, an increase in $FEV_1 \geq 15$ percent of baseline) or FVC as an acute response to a bronchodilator aerosol. Reversibility is necessary for the diagnosis of asthma, but an acute response may not be demonstrated in patients with asthma when their pulmonary function is extremely poor or when it is relatively normal. Although some reversibility may be demonstrated in patients who have chronic bronchitis or even emphysema, the degree is greater in asthmatics.

Reversibility to fully normal values is seen in younger patients with uncomplicated asthma. Many patients, particularly older ones, have persistently abnormal lung function, yet demonstrate episodic exacerbation of symptoms and response to treatment. The term "chronic asthmatic bronchitis" has been used to describe these patients. Reversibility is discussed in detail in Chapter 11.

RESTRICTIVE IMPAIRMENT

Definition

Total Lung Capacity Decreased

Restriction means *decrease in lung volume.* Ideally, this means decrease in TLC determined by body plethysmography, multiple-breath dilution, or a properly applied radiographic method. In restrictive impairments, the RV may be normal or decreased. If it is decreased proportionally to the VC (and therefore to the TLC), the lung volumes are said to be "miniaturized." If the RV is normal or decreased less than the VC, the RV/TLC is increased.

Total Lung Capacity and Residual Volume "Not Increased"

It is general experience that TLC is reduced far less often than VC in patients with ILD and that RV may be normal in patients with chest bellows and neuromuscular disorders. Therefore, in defining restrictive impairment, it may be more accurate to require that the TLC and RV be *not increased* rather than be "decreased."

The Limitation in Using the Vital Capacity to Define Restriction

A difficulty in applying the term restriction arises when the VC is the only lung volume measured. The VC, especially the FVC, is frequently reduced by air trapping in association with airways obstruction. Indeed, the greater the air trapping, the greater the reduction in VC and the less apparent the decrease in FEV_1/FVC or in flow rates, which are measured relative to the FVC. When air trapping is extreme and/or expiration is not sufficiently sustained, FEV_1/FVC will be normal.

Clues to Air Trapping When the FVC is Reduced

The interpreter of spirometry may utilize the following simple clues from the tests to detect air trapping when it is associated with a low FVC. The configuration of the MEVF and spirographic curves shows an obstructive concavity or even dynamic compression. A larger slow, or inspiratory VC than forced VC; or a negative forced ERV, ie, the tracing does not return to the resting baseline following the FVC maneuver are also clues. When flows and VC are both decreased, an equivalent or smaller decrease in flow suggests restrictive impairment, while a greater decrease in flow suggests an obstructive element. It is useful to bear in mind that the $FEF_{25-75\%}$ (in L/sec) is generally about 0.8 of the FVC (in L): the exact ratio for a particular individual is available from her predicted values for these two tests. A value below 0.65 indicates obstruction. Thus, an $FEF_{25-75\%}$ that is 50 percent of predicted does not mean obstruction or small airways obstruction if the VC is similarly decreased.

"Dynamic air trapping" (progressive increase in the end expiratory position) with the onset of the MVV maneuver (illustrated in Fig. 4-2) is a useful clue.

Of course, clinical and radiographic estimation of lung size, quality of breath sounds, wheezes, and other clinical findings are extremely useful in separating air trapping from a restrictive disorder.

Types of Restriction

Lung volumes are reduced and flows relatively maintained in several widely disparate types of disorder.

Diffuse Pulmonary Disease

Causes.   The same pattern of physiologic findings may be seen both in interstitial inflammatory or fibrotic disorders, and in alveolar filling processes. Certain findings, such as decrease in specific D_L or compliance, may be more characteristic of the interstitial disorders, which are far more common causes of chronic lung disease. Clinically, the distinction is not always easily made, and histologically, alveolar filling frequently accompanies interstitial inflammation and fibrosis. Thus, alveoli may be filled when desquamative changes accompany interstitial pneumonitis, and both alveolar luminal and interstitial inflammation may be seen in extrinsic allergic alveolitis. In reviewing lung biopsies at our weekly pathology conferences, we are often frustrated in our desire to classify cases neatly into one category or the other.

The etiologies of ILD are multiple. The tissue changes may be inflammatory, granulomatous, fibrotic, or neoplastic (lymphangitic carcinoma, lymphoma, or leukemic infiltration). The course of the disease may be rapid, proceding to death in weeks (as in postinfluenzal pulmonary fibrosis) or be stable for many years, as in various pneumoconioses.

Physiologic findings.   By definition, the VC is decreased. For reasons discussed above, the TLC may not be decreased but would be expected to decrease as the disease progresses. The following findings are characteristic of diffuse pulmonary disease: Increased recoil pressure and decreased static lung compliance; these are not generally performed clinical tests. Specific compliance is better preserved in alveolar filling diseases. Flows are often increased because of the increased recoil pressure of the lung and greater traction on the airways. We have noted that FEV_1/FVC and flows expressed as a ratio to FVC may be increased in patients with radiographically evident ILD who have normal lung volumes.

Alternately, flows may be reduced since inflammation and fibrosis are known to localize around airways in sarcoidosis and ILD of various etiologies.[18-20]

The MVV is generally normal until end stage. The air velocity index is high. Both D_LCO and D_L/V_A are generally reduced.

Reduction in PaO_2 on exercise is very common. Respiratory alkalosis is present for most of the course. Retention of CO_2 develops at end stage, when tidal volumes are so limited (≤ 250 cc) that dead space becomes a large part of the total ventilation.

Resection and Autopneumonectomy

When a lung or lobe is surgically resected, there is a decrease in lung volume more-or-less equivalent to the loss of tissue. The MVV and D_LCO decrease to a lesser extent, the former because the full VC is not needed to generate the MVV, and the latter because of increased perfusion and improved ventilation-perfusion balance in the remaining lung. A similar pattern may result from local inflammatory or necrotizing diseases (eg, tuberculosis), which result in more-or-less equal destruction of lung parenchyma, airways and vessels. This process has been likened to an "autopneumonectomy."

Chest Wall (or Chest Bellows) Disorders

Causes: skeletal deformities.   Kyphosis and/or scoliosis. Since Hippocrates, the "hunchback" has been known to be susceptible to breathing difficulties, cyanosis, and early death.

And in those cases where the gibbosity is above the diaphragm, the ribs do not expand properly . . . and the chest becomes sharp-pointed and not broad, and they become affected

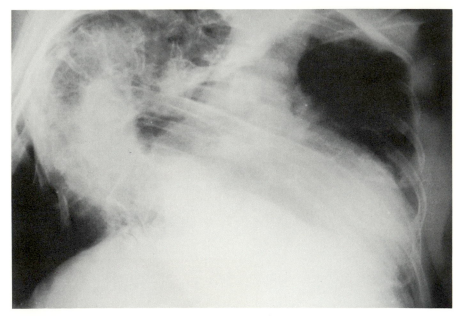

Fig. 10-4. Chest roentgenograph (PA projection) of an elderly patient with severe kypho-scoliosis. The extreme curvature and rotational deformity of the thoracic spine are typical of kyphoscoliosis at any age.

with difficulty of breathing and hoarseness; for the cavities which inspire and expire the breath do not attain their proper capacity. (Hippocrates, *On the Articulations,* translated by Frances Adams and quoted by Bergofsky, et al in 1959[21])

Kyphoscoliosis may be acquired following poliomyelitis or Pott's disease in childhood; congenital, associated with a wide variety of boney deformities involving fusion and absence of vertebrae[22] or "idiopathic," coming on during puberty. The striking deformity of the thorax is illustrated by the chest radiograph in Figure 10-4 and the photographs in Figure 10-5.

Morquio's syndrome.   This is an example of an hereditary skeletal disorder causing foreshortening of the chest cage without kyphoscoliosis.[23]

Thoracoplasty.   Thoracoplasty, previously used to treat cavitary disease, is an iatrogenic skeletal deformity of the chest cage.

Pleural Diseases.   Fibrothorax (fibrous pleuritis). A thick rind of scar tissue, often calcified, restricts expansion of the rib cage when it forms on the parietal pleura and/or expansion of the lung when on the visceral pleura (Fig. 10-6). Often both surfaces are involved and pleural symphysis results. Fibrous pleurisy is a well

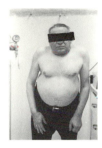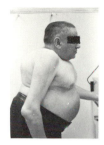

Fig. 10-5. Physical appearance of an elderly patient with kyphoscoliosis. Note foreshortening of the thoracic cage and "hunchback" deformity.

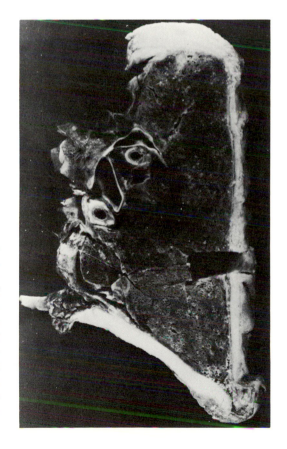

Fig. 10-6. Extensive pleural fibrosis and calcification from asbestos inhalation (post mortem). The lung parenchyma shows little evidence of fibrosis. The patient died at age 53 years in cardiorespiratory failure with CO_2 retention. [From Selikoff IJ. Asbestos-Associated Disease, in Maxcy-Rosenau, Public Health and Preventive Medicine [ed 11, Last JM (ED)]. New York. Appleton-Century-Crofts, 1980, p 574, with permission.]

known consequence of inhalation of asbestos fibers,[24] pyogenic empyema, tuberculous empyema (often following pneumothorax therapy) or traumatic hemothorax.

Case Presentation 10-2 is a 39-year-old Hispanic woman who contracted bilateral pulmonary tuberculosis at age seven years. She was treated with bilateral pneumothorax installations until she developed tuberculous empyema. Her activities had been limited her entire subsequent life because of dyspnea. Nevertheless, she completed law school and was a successful international attorney. At the time she was evaluated, she was dyspneic on walking an incline or a single flight of stairs. On physical examination of her chest, inspiratory expansion was not detectable and dullness was noted at both apices and bases. The chest film showed bilateral fibrocalcified pleura (Fig. 10-7). On pulmonary function testing (Table 10-3), VC, TLC, and MVV were markedly reduced consistent with restrictive chest wall impairment; FEV_1, $FEF_{25-75\%}$, and D_LCO_{SB} were proportionately reduced and were normal when corrected for the decreased volumes. The slight hypercapnia and hypoxemia were explained by hypoventilation (estimated ΔPA—a O_2 15 Torr).

Restrictive chest cage impairment as a result of fibrous pleurisy, with little or no interstitial fibrosis, is recognized to result from exposure to asbestos (Fig. 10-6). The pattern has been described as "entrapment of the lungs."[25] We have reported five patients with ventilatory failure resulting in hypercapnia,[26] one of whom is illustrated in Figure 10-8 and Table 10-4.

Unilateral fibrothorax of whatever etiology may have a deleterious effect on overall pulmonary function far in excess of its radiologic extent. This is illustrated by a patient with asbestos-induced pleural fibrosis, illustrated in Figure 10-9 and Table 10-5.

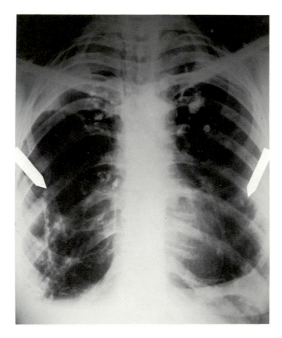

Fig. 10-7. (Case Presentation 10-2) Chest radiograph showing bilateral fibrocalcific pleurisy following pneumothorax therapy and tuberculous empyema at age 10. Note that the pleural thickening is especially prominent at the apices and costophrenic angles; the arrows indicate pleural calcification *en face*.

Table 10-3
Case Presentation 10-2, Bilateral
Fibrocalcific Pleurisy Long
After Pneumothorax Therapy in
a 39-Year-Old Hispanic Female
Nonsmoker, 160 cm, 47 kg

Lung Volumes	
VC (cc)	1050 (31%)
ERV	300
FRC (plet)	1860
TLC	2610 (55%)
RV	1560 (122%)
Spirometry and Flows	
FVC (cc)	1050 (31%)
FEV_1	890 (33%)
FEV_1/FVC	0.85
FEV_3FVC	1.00
PFR (L/sec)	3.1
$FEF_{25-75\%}$	0.82 (26%)
MVV (L/min)	33 (43%)
D_LCO_{SB} (cc/min/Torr)	9.53 (46%)
D_LCO/TLC_{SB}	3.81 (79%)
PaO_2, rest, Torr	78
$PaCO_2$, rest	45
pH	7.40

Pleural neoplasia. This is occasionally accompanied by a desmoplastic reaction having physiologic consequences similar to those of benign fibrothorax.

Large pleural or pericardial effusions. These may restrict chest wall function.

Increased abdominal pressure, obesity. Increased intraabdominal pressure, which limits diaphragmatic excursion, occurs with tense ascites and with obesity. In the latter, there is a linear increase in pressure with increasing weight; chest wall expansion may additionally be limited by the increased weight of soft tissues in the thorax.

Obesity may be defined as an increased body mass index (weight [kg]/height [M]²); a ratio of weight [kg]/height [cm] >0.4; or >125 percent of predicted body weight. When body mass index exceeds 30, mortality is increased.

The ERV is characteristically reduced, thus reducing the FRC, which is now smaller than the closing volume, resulting in perfusion of nonventilated alveoli during tidal breathing. Closing volume itself is not generally increased; closure occurs at the volume above RV at which it would be expected in the *normal* lung. Even before the relationship of closing volume to FRC was understood, it was noted

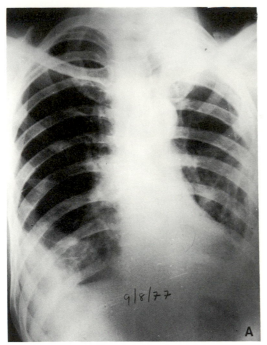
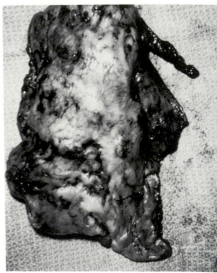

Fig. 10-8. (A) Chest radiograph showing bilateral fibrous pleurisy secondary to asbestos inhalation. The changes are most marked on the left side and at the right base. (B) Surgically resected pleura showing dense fibrosis and chronic inflammation. The pleura was up to 2 cm thick.

Table 10-4
Bilateral Fibrous Pleurisy
Secondary to Asbestos
Inhalation in a 52-Year-Old
Black Male Nonsmoker, 178
cm, 55 kg

Lung Volumes	
VC (cc)	1370 (28%)
ERV	470
FRC (plet)	2750
TLC	3650 (48%)
RV	2280 (85%)
Spirometry and Flows	
FVC (cc)	1370 (28%)
FEV_1	1090 (36%)
FEV_1/FVC	0.80
FEV_3/FVC	0.98
$DEF_{50\%}$ (L/sec)	3.13
$FEF_{75\%}$	0.98
MVV (L/min)	74 (74%)
PaO_2, rest, Torr	77
$PaCO_2$, rest	51
pH	7.40

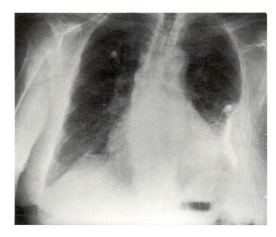

Fig. 10-9. Chest radiograph showing unilateral pleural fibrosis and calcification in a 59-year-old shipyard worker. Although the changes are confined to the lower half of the left pleura, the patient died in respiratory failure with CO_2 retention.

than an obese patient with an ERV less than 400 cc was likely to have severe hypoxemia.[27]

Physiologic Findings.   Most chest wall disorders are apparent *clinically*. Separation from restrictive impairment of the pulmonary type is therefore not difficult even though VC and TLC are reduced in both types. Physiologically, this distinction can generally be made on the following grounds:

The MVV is more likely to be reduced, often *para passu* with the decrease in VC.

The D_LCO is better maintained; D_L/VA is normal.

Retention of CO_2 develops at an earlier stage of disease. Indeed, chest cage disorders are classic causes of alveolar hypoventilation.

Table 10-5
Unilateral Fibrocalcific Pleurisy Causing
Respiratory Failure in a 60-Year-Old Black
Shipyard Worker Smoker, 174 cm, 95 kg

	6/76	4/78
Spirometry		
FVC (cc)	1965 (44%)	1720 (39%)
FEV_1	1640 (52%)	1530 (50%)
FEV_1/FVC	0.80	0.89
FEV_3/FVC	1.00	1.00
$FEF_{25-75\%}$ (L/sec)	2.57 (83%)	—
MVV (L/min)	57 (49%)	50 (44%)
PaO_2, rest, Torr		30–45*
$PaCO_2$, rest		70–90*

*Several determinations

The RV is least decreased of the lung volumes and may be normal. In other words, it is the *displaceable lung volumes* that are most decreased. Of 55 patients with idiopathic kyphoscoliosis, RV was normal, FRC was 79 percent, TLC 70 percent, and VC 61 percent of predicted.[28]

Reduced force generation: neuromuscular diseases. These are often classified under the chest bellows disorders but are fundamentally different in that the problem is not bellows *mobility* but bellows *activation*.

Causes. The responsible disorders include a large number of diseases of the central and peripheral nervous pathways leading to the diaphragm, intercostal muscles and abdominal muscles, as well as diseases of the motor endplates and muscles themselves. Most common are amyotrophic lateral sclerosis (ALS) also called motor neuron disease, traumatic transections of the spinal cord, Guillain-Barré syndrome (infectious polyneuropathy), myasthenia gravis, and various myopathies. The myopathies are commonly part of multisystem diseases that may involve the lung parenchyma and cause pulmonary restriction as well, such as dermatomyositis, polymyositis, and lupus erythematosus.

These diseases may follow an acute course (which may be reversible, as in Guillain-Barré syndrome) or an extremely protracted natural history. Both courses eventuate in ventilatory failure with CO_2 retention. Hypoxemia may be due to pure hypoventilation with a normal Δ A-a PO_2. Frequently, areas with low ventilation-perfusion ratios contribute to the hypoxemia as a result of inability to clear secretions, aspiration of mouth contents, and bronchopulmonary infection.

Before the advent of vaccines, poliomyelitis was the most widespread neuromuscular disease causing ventilatory failure. Much of the early development of mechanical ventilation was in response to polio epidemics in the decade after World War II.

Physiologic findings: Maximal respiratory pressures (forces). The earliest changes are likely to be a decrease in maximal inspiratory (P_{Imax} or P_{maxI}) and or expiratory pressure (P_{Emax} or P_{maxE}):[29,30] these are often summed to provide a single index of respiratory muscle strength.[31]

These pressures are easily measured by gauges or transducers.[30] P_{maxI} occurs close to RV, and P_{maxE} close to TLC; measurements are made at RV and TLC, respectively. Killian and Jones[32] measured P_{maxI} at FRC since this is the volume at which inspiration is normally initiated and it is not influenced by elastance of the lung or chest wall. Both P_{maxI} and P_{maxE} are sensitive to lung volume and corrections are necessary for P_{Imax} when RV exceeds 50 percent of predicted TLC and for P_{Emax} when TLC falls to less than 70 percent of its predicted value.[31] The most useful predicted equations are:

Normal values[30]
Equation 10-1a.

$$\text{Males: } P_{Imax} = 143 - 0.55A \text{ (cm } H_2O)$$
$$P_{Emax} = 268 - 1.03A$$

Equation 10-1b

$$\text{Females: } P_{Imax} = 104 - 0.51A$$
$$P_{Emax} = 170 - 0.53A$$

where A = age in years. Note that females have 65–70 percent of the strength of males and that strength decreases slightly with age (0.5–1.0 cm H_2O/year). When P_{maxI} is measured at FRC, the normal range is 66–120 cm H_2O.[32]

It is wise for each laboratory to confirm these normal values. In the author's laboratory, some normal subjects have been unable to achieve the values predicted above. The measurements test the combined strength of all the muscle groups. In the presence of neuromuscular disease with normal lungs, they appear to be the most sensitive of all simple tests.[29] In CAO, P_{Imax} is reduced because of increased RV causing unfavorable length-tension relationships, and possibly, weakness due to diaphragm atrophy. Chronic fatigue due to high resistive loads may occur but has not yet been demonstrated. It is conceivable that increased respiratory drive compensates for fatigue and that depression of the drive by, for example, oxygen allows the fatigue to manifest as respiratory failure.[33]

Although P_{Imax} and P_{Emax} are useful for the detection of respiratory impairment early in the course of neuuromuscular disorders, they are less useful for following the subsequent course, as illustrated in Table 10-6. This is precisely because these pressures are reduced to such an extent so early that further decreases are less obvious than decreases in spirometric measurements.

Spirometry. In ALS, spirometric results (including MVV) correlate better with prognosis than does the clinical neuromuscular examination. Ventilatory impairment manifested by a reduction in FVC (and MVV) as low as 50 percent of

Table 10-6
Masking of Airways Obstruction with Progression of Neuromuscular Disease in a 48-Year-Old Hispanic Woman With Amyotrophic Lateral sclerosis and Asthma, Nonsmoker, 163 cm, 55 kg

	5/82	8/82	12/82
Spirometry and Flows			
FVC (cc)	2710(67%)	2200(55%)	1300(34%)
FEV_1	1810(59%)	1720(56%)	1200(41%)
FEV_1/FVC	0.67	0.78	0.92
FEV_3/FVC	0.94	0.99	1.00
PFR (L/sec)	2.78	2.87	—
$FEF_{25-75\%}$	1.13(33%)	1.47(44%)	1.59(47%)
$FEF_{50\%}$	1.35	1.85	—
$FEF_{75\%}$	0.51	0.76	—
MVV (L/min)	47(49%)	47(49%)	—
P_I max (cm H_2O)	41(33%)	27(20%)	24(20%)
P_E max	54(24%)	25(11%)	16(7%)

predicted is often not appreciated by the patient or the physician. The lesson from this is to evaluate pulmonary function routinely in patients with neuromuscular disorders.

We have observed how the progressive loss of lung volumes masks coexisting CAO, as the FEV_1/FVC and flows become higher. This is illustrated in Table 10-6 which also shows rapid deterioration in 4 months. This is another important reason for performing pulmonary function testing as a routine in all patients with neuro-muscular disorders. Since airways obstruction is associated with an increased risk of pulmonary complications, it is important that it be detected.

Death in neuromuscular disorders is usually due to respiratory failure. Sequen-tial spirometry separates progressive impairment from a transient decrease in func-tion associated with intercurrent infection or aspiration. Precipitous irreversible declines in spirometric measurements may be seen; more rapid decline is noted as death approaches. An $FEV_1 \leq 0.7$ L presages CO_2 retention whether this level is reached rapidly or slowly.

Traumatic transection of the cervical cord. This catastrophe often strikes athletic young persons with normal lungs. Higher transections (C_{3-4}) result in bilat-eral diaphragmatic paralysis as well as loss of expiratory muscles. Because of the interdependence of the inspiratory and expiratory muscles, loss of ventilatory func-tion is only slightly less devastating in lower (C_{5-6}) lesions.

Botulism. Pulmonary complications include ventilatory failure and aspiration pneumonia. The VC was low in all 20 patients tested[34] and differentiated those patients who required ventilatory assistance (mean VC 34 percent of predicted) from those who did not (mean VC 55 percent of predicted) better than did the arterial gases; patients with a VC less than 33 percent of predicted always required ventilatory assistance. Because ventilatory failure was not identified clinically, it proceeded to respiratory arrest before being recognized. Improvement in respiratory function lagged behind improvement in cranial and somatic nerves.

Maximum voluntary ventilation. The MVV is a good overall index of neuro-muscular function.

Gas exchange. Gas exchange reflects alveolar ventilation and regional venti-lation–perfusion relationships. It is said to be well maintained in ALS even with severe spirometric impairment, so that arterial gas determinations may not be neces-sary in ambulatory patients.[35] When respiratory muscle strength is less than 30 percent, CO_2 retention is likely in myopathy.[36]

Diaphragmatic paralysis. Paralysis of the diaphragm may be recognized on clinical examination by paradoxical inward movement of the abdominal wall on inspiration, and on fluoroscopy by paradoxical upward displacement of the dia-phragm. Paradoxical motion is readily confirmed by inductance coils or magnetometers placed over the rib cage and abdomen. The transdiaphragmatic pressure gradient during a maximum inspiration is decreased, often to zero (normal >25 cm H_2O).

COMBINED (RESTRICTIVE-OBSTRUCTIVE) IMPAIRMENT

The VC is reduced as are the G_{aw}, FEV_1/FVC, flows, and MVV; the TLC and RV are not increased. Although this pattern can be defined only when full lung volumes are available, it is likely to be present in certain diseases and may be suspected from more limited testing.

Combined Impairment Due to a Single Disease Process

Chronic Granulomatous Diseases

Sarcoidosis and tuberculosis may cause endobronchial or peribronchial inflammation, granulomas, and fibrosis. The first large series demonstrating combined impairment in sarcoidosis was published by our group in 1974.[37] These patients had radiographic evidence of fibrosis such as hilar or diaphragmatic retraction, microcysts or bullae, which many authorities refer to as Stage IV. Of 16 patients, none had an increase in FRC, RV or TLC; 10 had a reduced VC, and 12 had evidence of airways obstruction. Although combined impairment is characteristic of this late stage of sarcoidosis with its extensive fibrosis, it may be seen in earlier stages and even when radiographic findings have cleared (Stage 0).

Cystic Fibrosis and Bronchiectasis

In these conditions, airways obstruction results from endobronchial and peribronchial inflammation and fibrosis, as well as endobronchial secretions. Restriction is attributable to the inflammatory and fibrotic changes in the lung.

Complicated Silicosis and Coal Workers' Pneumoconiosis

When progressive massive fibrosis supervenes (complicated pneumoconiosis), lung volume and indices of air flow are markedly decreased and there is progressive disability. It is illustrated by the pulmonary function tests shown in Table 10-7 and the chest radiograph seen in Figure 10-10. The patient had worked with a grinding wheel in a precious metal refinery. He was dyspneic on walking two blocks and had a productive cough.

Congestive Heart Failure

The VC has long been used to follow the course of congestive heart failure. Ries[38] noted a high correlation between VC and pulmonary capillary wedge pressure. Small airways obstruction as an early sign of interstitial pulmonary edema is well known.

Table 10-7

Combined Restrictive-Obstructive Impairment in Progressive Massive Fibrosis (Complicated Silicosis) in a 62-Year-Old Black Male Smoker, 160 cm, 61 kg

	5/81	5/83
Lung volumes		
VC (cc)	2040 (66%)	1760 (55%)
ERV	610	510
FRC (plet)	2750	2590
TLC	4180 (83%)	3840 (72%)
RV	2140 (109%)	2080 (101%)
Spirometry and Flows		
FVC (cc)	2040 (66%)	1760 (55%)
FEV_1	1200 (54%)	960 (42%)
FEV_1/FVC	0.59	0.54
FEV_3/FVC	0.85	0.78
PFR (L/sec)	1.86	1.93
$FEF_{25-75\%}$	0.68 (25%)	0.40 (15%)
R_{aw} (cm H_2O/L/sec)	4.3	—
MVV	54 (61%)	43 (47%)
D_LCO_{SB} (cc/min/Torr)		3.9 (20%)*
D_LCO/TLC_{SB}		0.93 (25%)*

*Predicted value for current smokers; result is 16 percent of predicted value for D_LCO_{SB} for nonsmokers.

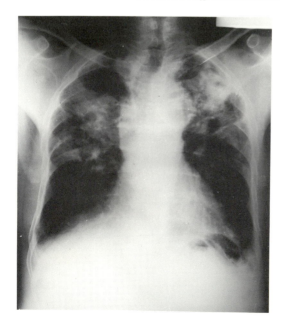

Fig. 10-10. Chest radiograph of a gold refiner showing progressive massive fibrosis secondary to silica. There are large, dense confluent infiltrates in both upper zones with central lucencies, as well as scattered 3–5 mm nodules.

Light and George[39] studied 28 patients with acute left ventricular failure not due to acute myocardial infarction. They reported typical combined impairment: mean FVC was 57 percent, FEV_1 48 percent, and $FEF_{25-75\%}$ 32 percent of predicted. Plethysmographic TLC was decreased (mean 82 percent of predicted).

Airways Function in Interstitial Lung Disease

Small Airways Obstruction

Histologic and physiologic evidence of small airways obstruction has been described in ILD of various etiologies.

Retention of fibers in respiratory bronchioles and an inflammatory response have been described in asbestos exposed individuals relatively early after onset of exposure and before evidence of diffuse pulmonary fibrosis. Limited studies of nonsmoking young asbestos workers have shown decreases in flows at low lung volume[40,41] and increases in closing volume.[42]

Overt Airways Obstruction

Physiologic evidence of overt airways obstruction is uncommon in ILD. However, airways obstruction not attributable to other causes is encountered in two uncommon types of ILD discussed below.

Histiocytosis-X (eosinophilic granuloma). Airways obstruction in this disease has been reviewed[43] and is illustrated by Case Presentation 10-3.

The diagnosis in this patient was made on open lung biopsy performed in 1969 because of diffuse reticulo-nodular infiltrates (Fig. 10-11). The prominent finding was aggregates of large histiocytes with various other cell types.

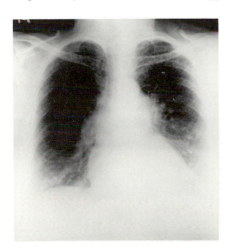 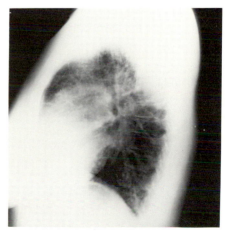

Fig. 10-11. (Case Presentation 10-3) Chest radiographs (PA and lateral) of a patient with eosinophilic granuloma diagnosed on open lung biopsy. Note large lung volume and diffuse small nodular-reticular infiltrate. The heart is enlarged and the hila prominent.

Table 10-8
Case Presentation 10-3, Severe Obstructive Impairment
in Eosinophilic Granuloma, 59-Year-Old White
Female Smoker, 159 cm, 68 kg

	3/79	7/79 (Corticosteroidoid Therapy)
Lung Volumes		
VC (cc)	2300(80%)	2410(84%)
ERV	610	820
FRC (plet)	4210	3820
TLC	5800(124%)	5410(118%)
RV	3600(204%)	3000(173%)
Spirometry and Flows		
FVC (cc)	2300(80%)	2100(73%)
FEV_1	1360(64%)	1300(61%)
FEV_1/FVC	0.59	0.62
$FEF_{25-75\%}$ (L/sec)	0.54(21%)	—
MVV (L/min)	55(74%)	64(87%)
D_LCO_{SB} (cc/min/Torr)	10.5(58%)*	7.4(41%)*
PaO_2, rest, Torr	59	48
$PaCO_2$, rest	42	50
pH, rest	7.40	7.47
PaO_2, minimal exercise	45	34

*Predicted values for current smokers; D_LCO_{SB} is 40 percent and 34 percent, respectively, of values for nonsmokers.

The patient's symptoms became progressive in 1975 and when she was admitted to The Mount Sinai Medical Center in 1979 she was dyspneic at rest and had lost 20 pounds. Physical examination revealed cyanosis, right ventricular heave and third heart sound, accentuated second pulmonic sound, diminished breath sounds, wheezing, basal crackles, and pretibial edema. On pulmonary function testing (Table 10-8), the VC was at the lower limits of normal, the RV was moderately increased, and the FEV_1/FVC and $FEF_{25-75\%}$ were decreased. The D_LCO_{SB} was considerably reduced despite a hematocrit of 57. The electrocardiogram showed right ventricular hypertrophy and right cardiac catheterization confirmed cor pulmonale (pulmonary artery pressure 120/55 Torr, mean 78; capillary wedge pressure 11 Torr, cardiac output 6.3 L/min). A large right ventricle and small left ventricle were demonstrated. The patient did not respond to corticosteroid or immunosuppressive therapy.

Lymphangioleiomyomatosis, a rare disease of young women involving hyperplasia of smooth muscles in pulmonary lymphatics, is associated with a reticulonodular infiltrate on chest roentgenogram, which is characteristic of ILD. However, lung function in this disorder is typically obstructive; flows are reduced. The TLC increases as the disease progresses. In five of six cases reported by Carrington,[44] FEV_1/FVC was ≤ 0.55.

Superimposition of Disease Processes

Since smoking is so prevalent a habit and asthma so common an illness, airways obstruction secondary to these causes is frequently noted in patients with any of the diseases causing restrictive impairment. Furthermore, bronchial distortion in parenchymal fibrosis or impaired clearance of secretions in chest wall disorders may predispose to airway infection and result in obstruction.

ISOLATED DIFFUSION DEFECT

Lung volumes, flows, and MVV are normal, but $D_L CO$ (and D_L/V_A) is reduced, often strikingly. There is frequently a fall in PaO_2 on exercise (including nonsteady-state "step-up" exercise).

Interstitial Lung Disease

Isolated diffusion defect is frequently seen in early stages (even with a normal chest radiograph) and is not uncommon even when disease is clinically manifest. In patients who have an isolated diffusion defect, we have often observed that flow-volume ratios such as FEV_1/FVC or $FEF_{50\%}/FVC$ are unusually high, which may reflect increased elastic recoil and traction on the airways.

Pulmonary Vascular Disease

The diffusion defect is accompanied by an increase in dead space ventilation.

Anemia and Abnormal Hemoglobin

These factors should be taken into consideration in the measurement of $D_L CO$ since they will lower its value (see Chapter 7).

RESPIRATORY CENTER UNRESPONSIVENESS

This is rare as the primary cause of respiratory failure but may be associated with other causes such as CAO, obesity, and obstructive sleep apnea. The essential findings in true central hypoventilation are hypercapnia and hypoxemia with normal lung volumes, flows, MVV, gas transfer, and muscle force. The alveolar–arterial difference for PO_2 may be normal, or increased in the presence of chronic bronchitis, retained secretions or obesity. Hypercapnia and hypoxemia reverse with voluntary hyperventilation or exercise.

Respiratory center responsiveness to CO_2 and/or hypoxia is diminished. The most available and standardized test of responsiveness is the CO_2 rebreathing method of Read.[45] Since pulmonary function is otherwise normal, a decrease in responsiveness cannot be attributed to end organ (airways, lung parenchyma, or chest wall) impairment.

ABNORMAL BLOOD GASES IN THE ABSENCE OF OTHER PULMONARY FUNCTION ABNORMALITIES

Hypoxemia

It is not unusual for the PaO_2 to be reduced, yet lung volumes, flows, D_LCO, MVV, and muscle force be normal, or for the widening of the alveolar-arterial difference for PO_2 and the degree of hypoxemia to be far greater than changes in other pulmonary function measurements.

Chest Bellows Disorders

This is characteristic of disorders that decrease chest wall mobility and/or increase abdominal pressure (especially obesity); the reduction in FRC results in airways closure occurring during tidal breathing.

Small Airways Obstruction

Small airways disease may not be apparent from the routine tests performed, yet cause sufficient ventilation–perfusion imbalance to result in hypoxemia. This is frequently the case in smokers, asymptomatic asthmatics, and patients with subclinical congestive heart failure.

ILD

In ILD, the exercise PaO_2 may be decreased even though the D_LCO and PaO_2 measured at rest are normal. Many clinicians include this exercise fall in PaO_2 as well as a decrease in D_LCO in the term "diffusion defect." Risk and coworkers noted that 26 of 94 (28 percent) patients with ILD and well preserved D_LCO_{SB} had significant increases in Δ A-a PO_2 on exercise.[46]

Venoarterial Shunt

If resting hypoxemia is severe in the absence of other abnormalities in pulmonary function, it may be a clue to a venoarterial shunt. This can then be measured by having the patient inhale 100 percent O_2, as discussed in Chapter 8.

Hypercapnia

Hypercapnia *by itself* does not occur as a result of pulmonary disease, unless the patient is breathing a high inspired O_2 concentration. It is always *associated with* (and usually preceded by) hypoxemia.

An elevation in CO_2 in the absence of other pulmonary function abnormalities may be the clue to respiratory center unresponsiveness (as discussed above). It is seen in patients on methadone maintenance.[47] Commonly, such an elevation is secondary to metabolic alkalosis from diuretic and/or corticosteroid therapy or vomiting. Since patients with chronic lung disease are frequently treated with these drugs and are likely to be troubled by vomiting, metabolic alkalosis is common and may "mask" the expected respiratory acidosis. This may not present a problem to the clinician when the underlying predisposition to hypoventilation is known. However, when the history is not available, the patient may be presumed to have metabolic alkalosis from her blood gas findings without recognition of the risk of further CO_2 retention, especially when oxygen or sedation is employed. We have proposed inhalation of 100 percent O_2 for 15 minutes to demonstrate an underlying respiratory acidosis in patients presenting with apparent metabolic alkalosis.[48] Respiratory acidosis developed in 19 of 32 patients (59 percent) who had associated CAO or chest bellows disorders but in only one of 10 whose metabolic alkalosis was due to intensive diuretic therapy of congestive heart failure or steroid therapy of ILD. Hypoxemia was not useful in separating patients who were at risk for respiratory acidosis, since it was frequent in both groups of patients.

A $PaCO_2 \geq 54$ Torr seldom results from metabolic alkalosis alone and generally indicates that ventilatory failure is present, whatever the pH may be.

References

1. Weibel ER. Morphometry of the human lung. Heidelberg. Springer Verlag, 1963
2. Horsfield K, Cumming G. Morphology of the bronchial tree in man. J Appl Physiol 24:373–383, 1968
3. Macklem PT, Mead J. Resistance of central and peripheral airways measured by a retrograde catheter. J Appl Physiol 22:395–401, 1967
4. Van Brabandt H, Cauberghs M, Verbeken E, et al. Partitioning of pulmonary impedance in excised human and canine lungs. J Appl Physiol: Respir Environ Ex 55:1733–1742, 1983
5. Hoppin FG Jr, Green M, Morgan MS. Relationship of central and peripheral airway resistance to lung volume in dogs. J Appl Physiol: Respirat Environ Ex 44:728–737, 1978
6. Macklem PT, Thurlbeck WM, Fraser RG. Chronic obstructive disease of small airways. Ann Intern Med 74:167–177, 1971
7. Hogg JC, Macklem PT, Thurlbeck WM. Site and nature of airway obstruction in chronic obstructive lung disease. N Engl J Med 278:1355–1360, 1968
8. Jayamanne DS, Epstein H, Goldring RM. Flow-volume curve contour in COPD: Correlation with pulmonary mechanics. Chest 77:749–757, 1980
9. Laurell CB, Eriksson S. The electrophoretic alpha 1-globulin pattern of serum in alpha 1-antitrypsin deficiency. Scand J Lab Invest 15:132–140, 1963
10. Eriksson S. Studies in α_1-antitrypsin deficiency. Acta Med Scand (suppl 432) 1–85, 1965
11. Schwartz HR. Hypocomplementemic urticarial vasculitis: Association with chronic obstructive pulmonary disease. Mayo Clin Proc 57:231–238, 1982

12. Turton CW, Williams G, Green M. Cryptogenic obliterative bronchiolitis in adults. Thorax 36:805–810, 1981

13. Seggev J, Mason UG III, Worthen S, et al. Bronchiolitis obliterans. Report of three cases with detailed physiologic studies. Chest 83:169–174, 1983

14. Epler GR, Colby TV, McLoud TC, et al. Bronchiolitis obliterans organizing pneumonia. N Engl J Med 312:152–158, 1985

15. Epler GR, Snider GL, Gaensler EA, et al. Bronchiolitis and bronchitis in connective tissue disease. JAMA 242:528–532, 1979

16. Ralph DD, Springmeyer SC, Sulivan KM, et al. Rapidly progressive air-flow obstruction in marrow transplant recipients. Possible association between obliterative bronchiolitis and chronic graft-versus-host disease. Am Rev Respir Dis 129:641–644, 1984

17. Roca J, Granena A, Rodriguez-Roisin R, et al. Fatal airway disease in an adult with chronic graft-versus-host disease. Thorax 33:77–78, 1982

18. Ostrow D, Cherniack RM. Resistance to air flow in patients with diffuse interstitial lung disease. Am Rev Respir Dis 108:205–210, 1973

19. Crystal RG, Fulmer JD, Roberts WC, et al. Idiopathic pulmonary fibrosis. Clinical, histologic, radiographic, physiologic, scintigraphic, cytologic and biochemical aspects. Ann Intern Med 85:769–788, 1976

20. Levinson RS, Metzger LF, Stanley N, et al. Airway function in sarcoidosis. Am J Med 62:51–59, 1977

21. Bergofsky EH, Turino GM, Fishman AP. Cardiorespiratory failure in kyphoscoliosis, Medicine 38:263–317, 1959

22. Baga N, Chusid EL, Miller A. Pulmonary disability in the Klippel-Feil syndrome (a study of 2 siblings). Clin Orthoped Rel Res 67:105–110, 1969

23. Buhain WJ, Rammohan G, Berger HW. Pulmonary function in Morquio's disease: A study of two siblings. Chest 68:41–45, 1975

24. Navratil M, Dobias J. Development of pleural hyalinosis in long term studies of persons exposed to asbestos dust. Environ Research 6:455–472, 1973

25. Wright PH, Hanson A, Kreel L, et al. Respiratory function changes after asbestos pleurisy. Thorax 35:31–36, 1980

26. Miller A, Teirstein AS, Selikoff I. Ventilatory failure due to asbestos pleurisy. Am J Med 75:911–919, 1983

27. Holley HS, Milic-Emili J, Becklake MR, et al. Regional distribution of pulmonary ventilation and perfusion in obesity. J Clin Invest 46:475–481, 1967

28. Kafer ER. Idiopathic scoliosis: Mechanical properties of the respiratory system and the ventilatory response to carbon dioxide. J Clin Invest 55:1153–1163, 1975

29. Black LF, Hyatt RE. Maximal static respiratory pressures in generalized neuromuscular disease. Am Rev Respir Dis 103:641–650, 1971

30. Black LF, Hyatt RE. Maximal respiratory pressures: Normal values and relationship to age and sex. Am Rev Resp Dis 99:696–702, 1969

31. Ringqvist T. The ventilatory capacity in healthy subjects: An analysis of causal factors with special reference to the respiratory forces. Scand J Clin Lab Invest 18(suppl 88):5–179, 1966

32. Killian KJ, Jones NL. The use of exercise testing and other methods in the investigation of dyspnea. Clin Chest Med 5:99–108, 1984

33. Rochester DF, Arora NS, Braun NMT, et al. The respiratory muscles in chronic obstructive pulmonary disease. Bull Europ Physiopath Resp 15:951–975, 1979

34. Schmidt-Nowara WW, Samet JM, Rosario PA. Early and late pulmonary complications of botulism. Arch Intern Med 143:451–456, 1983

35. Fallat RJ, Jewitt B, Bass M, et al. Spirometry in amyotrophic lateral sclerosis. Arch Neurol 36:74–80, 1979

36. Braun NMT, Rochester DF. Muscular weakness and respiratory failure. Am Rev Respir Dis 119(Part 2):123–125, 1979

37. Miller A, Teirstein AS, Jackler I, et al. Airway function in chronic pulmonary sarcoidosis with fibrosis. Am Rev Respir Dis 109:179–189, 1974

38. Ries AL, Gregoratos G, Friedman PJ, et al. Lung volumes in assessment of left heart failure. Am Rev Respir Dis 123(Part 2):A103, 1981

39. Light RW, George RB. Serial pulmonary function in patients with acute heart failure. Arch Intern Med 143:429–433, 1983

40. Harless KW, Watanabe S, Renzetti AD Jr. The acute effects of chrysotile asbestos exposure on lung function. Environ Research 16:360–372, 1978

41. Rodriguez-Roisin R, Merchant JEM, Cochrane GM. Maximal expiratory flow-volume (MEVF) curves in workers exposed to asbestos. Resp 39:158, 1980

42. DiMenza L, Ruff F, Bignon J. Obstruction des voies aeriennes peripheriques au cours de l'exposition professionelle a l'amiante. Ann d'Anat Path 21:261–268, 1976

43. Friedman PJ, Liebow AA, Sokoloff J. Eosinophilic granuloma of the lung. Clinical aspects of primary pulmonary histiocytosis in the adult. Medicine 60:385–396, 1981

44. Carrington CB, Cugell DW, Gaensler EA, et al. Lymphangioleiomyomatosis. Physiologic-pathologic-radiologic correlations. Am Rev Respir Dis 116:977–998, 1977

45. Read DJC. A clinical method for assessing the ventilatory response to carbon dioxide. Australas Ann Med 16:20–32, 1966

46. Risk C, Epler GR, Gaensler EA. Exercise alveolar-arterial oxygen pressure difference in interstitial lung disease. Chest 85:69–74, 1984

47. Marks CE Jr, Goldring RM. Chronic hypercapnia during methadone maintenance. Am Rev Respir Dis 108:1088–1093, 1973

48. Miller A, Teirstein AS, Duberstein J, et al. Use of oxygen inhalation in evaluation of respiratory acidosis in patients with apparent metabolic alkalosis. Am J Med 45:513–519, 1968

Part IV

Special Applications

11

Bronchodilator and Provocational Tests

Albert Miller

Bronchodilator Response
  Agents
  What is a Positive Response?
    Conventional Definition
    Statistical Definition
    Volume Response versus Flow Response
  Isovolume Comparison of Flows
  Uses of the BD Response
    In the Diagnosis of Asthma
    As a Guide to Therapy
    In Prognosis
Provocational Response
  Agents
    Pharmacologic Agents
    Specific Antigens
    Workplace Exposure
    Nonpharmacologic, Nonimmunologic Challenge
  Aerosol Inhalation Schedules
  Definition of a Positive Test
  Clinical Applications of Tests for Bronchial Hyperreactivity
    The Diagnosis of Asthma
    The Diagnosis of Atypical Asthma
    Other Causes of Hyperreactivity
    Selection of Patients for Treatment with Beta Blockers

PULMONARY FUNCTION TESTS: A   ISBN 0-8089-1764-4   Copyright © 1987 by Grune & Stratton
GUIDE FOR THE STUDENT AND HOUSE OFFICER   All rights of reproduction in any form reserved.

Repeat pulmonary function testing after use of agents that reverse or induce bronchoconstriction provides valuable information that cannot be obtained in other ways.

BRONCHODILATOR RESPONSE

Agents

The BD generally used is an aerosol adrenergic drug that may be B_2-specific and therefore affect predominantly bronchial smooth muscle (eg, albuterol). Anticholinergic aerosols also induce BD in asthmatics and may be more potent than adrenergic agonists in chronic bronchitis (see below).

The aerosol may be delivered by a propellant-powered metered-dose cartridge or by an air compressor. For patients otherwise unable to inhale the aerosol, it may be given by mask. Beta-agonists and atropine may be used parenterally when the patient is unable to inhale an aerosol.

What is a Positive Response?

Conventional Definition

The conventional definition of a positive response is an increase in FEV_1 *or* FVC ≥ 15 percent compared with the pre-BD value. As with other tests expressed as a percentage change from baseline, the absolute value of the change and of the baseline must be taken into consideration. The FEV_1 or FVC must increase at least 200 cc for a percentage increase ≥ 15 percent to be considered significant.

When BD-response is plotted against baseline spirometric values in patients whose asthma is undergoing exacerbation and remission, an inverted U-shaped curve results[1] (Fig. 11-1). The least improvement is seen when baseline values are lowest (often due to diffuse mucus plugging) or highest (relatively normal bronchial tone). On the other hand, it is not unusual for asthmatics with normal values for FVC and FEV_1 to show considerable increases post-BD, even ≥ 15 percent.

Statistical Definition

Several investigators have measured the BD response in *normal subjects* and calculated 95 percent confidence intervals similar to these reported by Sourk and Nugent[2]: 5.2 percent change from baseline for FVC, 10.5 percent for FEV_1, and 49 percent for $FEF_{25-75\%}$. Confidence intervals in *patients*, who have greater intrasubject variability, have been calculated based on changes after *placebo* inhalations. Shown in Table 11-1, these are very similar to the conventional definitions of BD response.

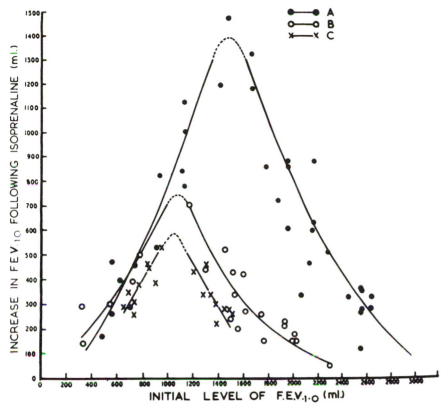

Fig. 11-1. Increase in FEV₁ after BD, plotted against the baseline value; repeated measurements in three patients. Note that increases are least when baseline values are lowest or highest. [From Hume KM, Gandevia B. Forced expiratory volume before and after isoprenaline. Thorax 12:277, 1957 with permission.]

Table 11-1
Ninety-five Percent Confidence
Limits for Changes in Spirometry
After Placebo Inhalations in Patients

	Absolute Change	Percent Change
FVC L	0.340	14.9
FEV₁ L	0.178	12.3
FEV₁/FVC	0.09	16.7
FEF$_{25-75\%}$ L/sec	—	45.1

From Sourk RL and Nugent KM. Bronchodilator testing: Confidence intervals derived from placebo inhalations. Am Rev Resp Dis 128:155, 1983, with permission.

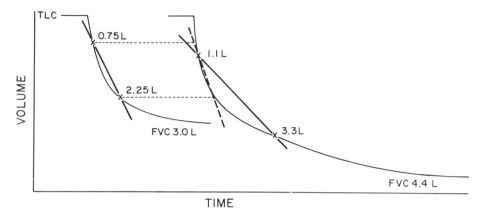

Fig. 11-2. Isovolume adjustment of FEF$_{25-75\%}$. The spirometric tracings are matched at TLC. The initial (in this case, pre-BD) 25 percent and 75 percent points are carried over to the second (in this case, post-BD) curve. Flows are therefore measured over the same volume from TLC in both tracings. Note that when volume-adjusted, the FEF$_{25-75\%}$ is slightly increased post-BD (dashed line) while it is decreased when measured relative to the larger post-BD FVC (heavy line).

Volume Response versus Flow Response

Some patients show a predominant increase in FVC with lesser change in FEV$_1$. Ramsdell and Tisi[3] noted that 41 percent of their asthmatic patients whose pulmonary function improved with a BD aerosol were such "volume responders," whose FEV$_1$/FVC fell compared with baseline. The volume responders had greater baseline airways obstruction and air trapping.

Isovolume Comparison of Flows

If flow rates are evaluated post-BD, these must be at the same volume as (isovolume to) the baseline flows. Since it may be assumed that TLC does not change markedly, flows can be compared at the same expired volume from full inspiration. This is illustrated in Figure 11-2 for FEF$_{25-75\%}$ and Figure 11-3 for FEF$_{50\%}$ and FEF$_{75\%}$. If FEF$_{50\%}$ pre-BD occurs after 2L have been expired, comparison post-BD should be at 2L from full inspiration. Since FVC often increases post-BD, so that the FEF$_{50\%}$ of the post-BD effort is at a volume greater than 2L from TLC, *comparison at isovolume will generally make any increase in flow more evident.* Quite often, with a large increase in FVC, instantaneous or mean flows measured relative to the actual post-BD FVC (ie, not isovolume) will be *lower* than the pre-BD values because they are measured at a considerably lower lung volume[4]; this is seen in Figure 11-2. For the same reason, FEV$_1$/FVC is often lower post-BD despite increases in both FEV$_1$ and FVC (eg, the "volume responders" described above).

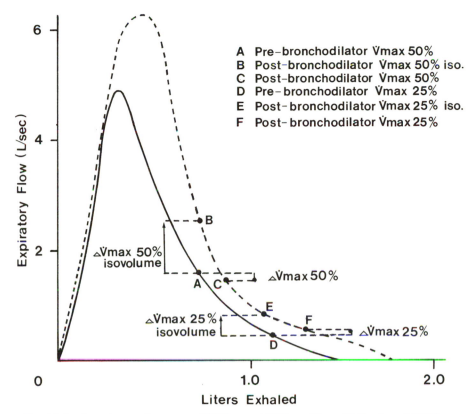

Fig. 11-3. Isovolume adjustment of FEF$_{50\%}$ and FEF$_{75\%}$. The solid line is an MEFV curve *pre*-BD and the dashed line a curve *post*-BD. Curves are matched at TLC. Note that the isovolume flows in the post-BD curve are larger than the flows relative to FVC. In fact, the non-adjusted FEF$_{50\%}$ is lower than the pre-BD value. [From Lorber DB, Kaltenborn W, Burrows B. Responses to isoproterenol in a general population sample. Am Rev Resp Dis 118:856, 1978, with permission.]

It has been suggested that when flows are compared isovolume, an increase in FEF$_{25-75\%}$ or FEF$_{50\%}$ ≥ 30% is significant.[5]

Uses of the BD Response

In the Diagnosis of Asthma

Reversibility is a *sine qua non* of asthma. Many young asthmatics will normalize their spirometric values post-BD. However, a positive response does not establish the clinical diagnosis of asthma since an element of reversibility may be observed in other obstructive diseases. Therefore, additional clinical and physiologic data are necessary. The differential diagnosis of airways obstruction and the role played by BD-testing are discussed in Chapter 10.

An asthmatic patient may not show a positive response each time he is tested. An exacerbation associated with diffuse mucus plugging will often not respond (and may interfere with delivery of the aerosol) while a state of remission with normal baseline function may show little percentage change (Figure 11-1). Kanner[6] confirmed a negative correlation between BD response and pre-BD FEV_1. It is therefore recommended that, in a patient with overt airways obstruction, a trial of BD therapy including steroids be employed before reversibility is ruled out.[7]

Several investigators have noted a greater response to anticholinergic agents (aerosol ipratropium bromide, atropine methonitrate or glycopyrrolate, or oral atropine sulfate) than to adrenergic BD drugs in patients with chronic bronchitis, consistent with a state of vagotonia. Since ipratropium is poorly absorbed on inhalation, it does not affect mucus production or clearance or induce tremor, tachycardia, glaucoma, or bladder neck obstruction.[8]

As a Guide to Therapy

While many clinicians will utilize BD drugs to treat airways obstruction even when a positive response is not demonstrated, such therapy is unlikely to be of benefit when the BD-response remains consistently negative. Response to BD predicts benefit from oral theophylline[9] as well as from adrenergic agents. Continued absence of response in patients with strong clinical evidence of asthma may suggest earlier or more intensive use of steroids.

Although a course of corticosteroid therapy may enable previously unresponsive patients to show a positive acute BD response, there is, on the whole, a relationship between the acute response to BD and the subacute response to steroids. Mandella[10] described the effects of two weeks of high dose methylprednisolone on the FEV_1 of 46 patients with stable CAO. Eight patients showed a marked increase. Their only distinguishing characteristic was a greater response to aerosol BD (25 percent versus 13 percent). Patients who demonstrated less than a 10 percent acute response were unlikely to benefit from steroids.

The relationship of the acute BD response to the provocational response in patients with CAO is of interest. Ramsdell et al[11] studied 22 patients with stable "chronic obstructive bronchitis" who did not show an acute BD response. All demonstrated marked hyperreactivity on methacholine challenge. The authors suggested that chronic BD therapy was indicated in these patients as well. It is possible that a course of steroids would have rendered some of them acutely BD-responsive.

In Prognosis

In using spirometric results to evaluate pulmonary reserve in CAO, reserve and therefore prognosis correlate better with post-BD values. Similarly, ability to withstand surgery should be assessed post-BD.

The BD response helps predict the annual rate of decline in FVC and FEV_1 in patients with CAO: the greater the responsiveness, the more rapid the decline.[6]

Similar relationships have been reported for airway responsiveness assessed by bronchoprovocation (see below).

PROVOCATIONAL RESPONSE

Agents

Pharmacologic Agents

Methacholine chloride or mecholyl™ is a cholinergic drug that stimulates acetylcholine receptors on bronchial smooth muscle cells; it can be blocked by atropine and counteracted by adrenergic bronchodilators. Although methacholine and histamine provide similar information, methacholine is more widely used because patients are more reactive to it, it does not induce acquired unresponsiveness seen occasionally with histamine,[12] and it brings about fewer side effects at higher dosage.[13] Patients with bradyarrhythmias or frequent vasovagal reactions and others at risk from a cholinergic drug should not be tested.

Despite reductions in G_{aw}, FEV_1, and flows and increases in RV and TLC induced by pharmacologic aerosols, gas exchange is not greatly impaired.

Pharmacologic agents will affect lung function in all subjects at sufficient dose (>25 mg/cc). Malo and coinvestigators[14] evaluated provocative concentrations of methacholine in 100 normal nonsmokers. Only three showed a 20 percent fall in FEV_1 at 8 mg/ml and eight at 16 mg/ml. There was thus a rather small overlap into the range of response which may be considered hyperreactive. Serial measurements of PFR did not suggest asthma in these subjects.

Specific Antigens

These may provoke an immediate (type I immunologic) response measurable as a fall in FEV_1 within 10–30 minutes or a delayed obstructive response observable after 6–12 hours. Several antigens have the potential of inducing both immediate type I and later type III responses in which physiologic tests (fall in VC, D_LCO, and lung compliance), clinical findings (fever and rales), and radiographic patterns (alveolar filling infiltrates) suggest parenchymal involvement. In contrast, pharmacologic agents produce only immediate responses (within 90 seconds to 5 minutes), which return to baseline in less than 90 minutes or respond readily to BD drugs.

Workplace Exposure

This form of challenge was comprehensively reviewed by Pepys and Hutchcroft.[15] It may be the only way to confirm an occupational or avocational cause for respiratory symptoms. Reproducing the workplace exposure in the laboratory (eg, by mixing the actual ingredients or subjecting them to the same processes) is often necessary. Testing at the actual work site preworkshift and postworkshift is another example of this approach, much used to evaluate such exposures as cotton dust and toluene-di-isocyanate (TDI).

Nonpharmacologic, Nonimmunologic Challenge

Inhalation of aerosols of hypertonic saline or distilled water. These have been used to detect bronchial hyperreactivity.[16,17] Hogg and Eggleston[18] have recently reviewed the effects of hypo-osmolar and hyperosmolar aerosols on airway tone and cough. Asthmatic airways adapt poorly to "osmotic stress." The basic defect may be an inability (by the epithelium) "to control the osmolarity and ion concentration of the fluid lining the airway surface."

Exercise and voluntary hyperventilation. These are widely used in children. The mechanism for bronchoconstriction includes loss of heat and water (see below), consistent with the clinical observation that swimming in an indoor pool is the least likely form of exercise to induce asthma in susceptible subjects. Exercise is associated with a greater number of false-negative responses than are pharmacologic aerosols.[19] It is discussed more fully in Chapter 12.

Isocapnic hyperventilation with cold air. The response to isocapnic hyperventilation with cold air, expressed as the respiratory heat exchange in Kcals/min required to reduce the FEV_1 by 10 percent, is similar to the response to methacholine expressed as the concentration causing a decrease in FEV_1 of 20 percent.[20] The test has been "simplified" by generating subfreezing air in an alcohol or acetone bath, which contains dry ice, while maintaining eucapnia by adding 1–2 L/min of 100 percent CO_2 to the inspired air. Such a challenge did not affect the lung function of normal subjects while it reduced the FEV_1 of asthmatics by 32.7 percent.[21] There was no overlap between normal and asthmatic subjects in this study, although responses to cold air have been reported in normal subjects.[22]

Dry air. Heat loss from the airways is generally linked to water loss, suggesting that a change in epithelial osmolarity may be important in inducing bronchoconstriction, as discussed above. Asthmatic subjects bronchoconstrict when breathing warm, dry air, which minimizes cooling but still causes water loss.[23] Eucapnia has been maintained during hyperventilation by breathing a single concentration of CO_2 (5 percent) in compressed air.[24]

Combination of factors. Several factors may induce bronchoconstriction in concert when one of them by itself does not, eg, exercise with cold or dry air in subjects who do not respond to exercise alone.

Aerosol Inhalation Schedules

In the standard protocol,[25] the subject is exposed to progressively larger doses of methacholine, histamine or antigen after he is tested with the diluent alone. Corrao[26] used a simple two-step challenge beginning with one breath of the highest concentration (25 mg/ml) and going on to an additional four breaths of the same concentration. With this, he demonstrated the usefulness of methacholine to detect bronchial hyperreactivity as the etiology of chronic cough. If one concentration of methacholine or histamine were to be selected in order to simplify and speed testing, it should be 8–10 mg/ml. This best separates normal from asthmatic subjects.[14,27]

Definition of a Positive Test

Most authorities agree on a fall in $FEV_1 \geq 20$ percent of the post-diluent baseline as a positive test. Other suggested end points are falls in $FVC \geq 10$ percent, $PFR \geq 20$ percent, $FEF_{25-75\%}$ and $FEF_{50\%} \geq 25-30$ percent, or specific $G_{aw} \geq 35-40$ percent or an increase in $FRC \geq 25$ percent.[25,28] Flows should be measured isovolume (see above). The different end points reflect the greater increase in SG_{aw} seen in normal subjects.

A positive test may be defined as evidence of airways obstruction at a dose of provocational agent which does not produce obstruction in normal individuals. In clinical use, this provocational concentration (PC) or provocational dose (PD; for FEV_1, this is the PD_{20}) is expressed as the *lowest actual concentration at which a positive* response occurs. This can be estimated by interpolating between the last two concentrations inhaled.

Clinical Applications of Tests for Bronchial Hyperreactivity

The Diagnosis of Asthma

A positive response to methacholine establishes that bronchial hyperreactivity (the syndrome of "twitchy airways") is present, and is consistent with the concept of autonomic imbalance in asthma.

In the absence of factors cited below, bronchial hyperreactivity may be considered part of the spectrum of asthma. A patient who once demonstrates an abnormal response will generally demonstrate such a response when tested later. It was at first believed that her dose-response curve would remain constant, with a variability of one dilution. It has since been shown that the provocational dose of patients with chronic allergic asthma can increase markedly when they are placed in an environment in which allergen levels are very low (Fig. 11-4). Decreased reactivity has also been demonstrated after specific hyposensitization.[29]

A provocational test is the most practical way to confirm a diagnosis of asthma when pulmonary function tests are normal or nonspecific minor changes are detected (eg, small airways obstruction). In addition, the magnitude of response to challenge correlates with the severity of asthma.[30-32]

The Diagnosis of Atypical Asthma

The patient with a positive provocational test may be free of symptoms or may have symptoms (now or in the past) which are not characteristic of asthma, such as

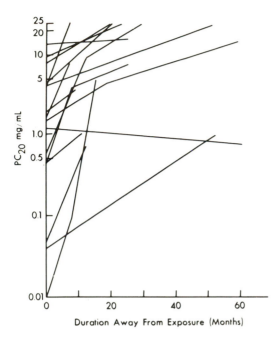

Fig. 11-4. Serial bronchial responses to methacholine expressed as PC_{20} for FEV_1 at intervals free from exposure in 16 workers with asthma secondary to Western red cedar. All became asymptomatic after they left the industry. Note the increase in PC_{20} with increased duration away from exposure in all workers. In eight workers, the PC returned to normal. [From Chan-Yeung M. Immunologic and nonimmunologic mechanisms in asthma due to western red cedar (*Thuja plicata*). J Allergy Clin Immunol 70:35, 1982, with permission.]

persistent cough or dyspnea without wheezing. Provocational testing should be part of the evaluation of persistent cough and of episodic dyspnea of no other apparent etiology. A negative response in a patient with symptoms virtually rules out bronchial hyperreactivity as their cause.

Other Causes of Hyperreactivity

Atopy, allergic rhinitis, and hypersensitivity pneumonitis. These are associated with a greater frequency of provocational response even when unaccompanied by evidence of asthma.

Acute respiratory infections. Hyperreactivity can persist for up to three months, and is probably related to damage to the respiratory mucosa and irritation of sensory receptors. This state helps explain the prolonged cough of which patients frequently complain following acute respiratory infection.

Recent Immunization (Influenza, Rubella).

Chronic bronchitis. The frequency of a positive response to pharmacologic agents is of interest in chronic bronchitis. As noted above, Ramsdell and co-workers[11] reported that all 22 patients they studied showed hyperreactivity to methacholine. The high frequency of bronchial hyperreactivity in chronic bronchitis was confirmed by Bahous.[33] Two-thirds of their non-BD-responsive chronic bronchitics had a $PD_{20} < 16$ mg/ml.

Yan[34] recently evaluated bronchial hyperreactivity in subjects with CAO versus those with asthma. Almost half the subjects with CAO demonstrated hyperreactivity to histamine. Their hyperreactivity differed from that in asthma, having a higher PD_{20} and a strong correlation between FEV_1/FVC and PD_{20}.

Thus, provocational testing may not be useful to separate individual patients with clinical asthma from those with chronic bronchitis, unless the response is negative.

Other pulmonary diseases. About 50 percent of patients with sarcoidosis manifest increased reactivity, regardless of stage, both in our experience and in that of others.[35] A high percentage of patients with cystic fibrosis show positive responses.[19]

Nevertheless, when another disease of the lungs is present or suspected, a positive test often indicates that symptoms are caused by bronchial hyperreactivity.

This is illustrated by Case Presentation 11-1, a 62-year-old woman who underwent left radical mastectomy in 1962, radiotherapy postoperatively and in 1972 for local recurrence, and multiple courses of chemotherapy since 1976 for extensive bone metastasis. The lungs were clear on physical examination and the chest film was negative. The recent onset of dyspnea in this patient, without previous respiratory symptoms or disease and without wheezing, strongly suggested lymphangitic carcinoma or a drug-induced interstitial pneumonitis. Pulmonary function is shown in Table 11-2. The normal D_LCO and lung volumes were evidence to the contrary and the positive response to methacholine incriminated bronchial hyperreactivity as the cause of her dyspnea. The patient could not tolerate bronchodilator medication. However, bronchial hyperreactivity was borne out by the observations over the next eight months that the dyspnea was now intermittent and that the D_LCO, lung volumes and chest film remained normal.

On several occasions in our experience, pulmonary vascular and/or interstitial involvement was strongly suspect in dyspneic patients with underlying connective tissue disease and negative chest films. Lung biopsy was considered. Relatively normal pulmonary function (especially D_LCO) and positive methacholine tests incriminated bronchial hyperreactivity, which was confirmed by response to BD therapy and nonprogression of disease on follow-up.

Pulmonary damage in childhood. Various injuries in childhood may increase bronchial reactivity permanently: Corrective surgery for congenital tracheo-esophageal fistula,[36] bronchopulmonary dysplasia following assisted ventilation for neonatal respiratory distress,[37] foreign body aspiration,[38] near drowning.[39]

Smoking. Various irritants increase the excitability of receptors in the airways and therefore induce bronchial hyperreactivity. Among these is tobacco smoke. Several investigators have reported hyperreactivity in current smokers, which is independent of atopy.[40-43]

The mechanism for the increase in bronchial reactivity induced by smoking may be epithelial injury or increased permeability exposing subepithelial irritant

Table 11-2

Case Presentation 11-1. Bronchial Hyperreactivity in a Patient
Thought to Have Lymphangitic Carcinoma of the Breast,
62-year-old White Female Nonsmoker, 152 cm, 61 kg*

	11/82	Methacholine 10 mg/cc	6/83
Lung Volumes			
VC (cc)	2580(102%)	2310, $\Delta = -17\%$	2700(107%)
ERV	1120	520	1300
FRC (plet)	2820	3190, $\Delta = +13\%$	2950
RV	1700(135%)	2670, $\Delta = +57\%$	1650(131%)
TLC	4680(123%)	5040, $\Delta = +8\%$	4350(115%)
Spirometry and Flows			
FVC (cc)	2370(94%)	2070, $\Delta = -13\%$	2700(107%)
FEV_1	1940(105%)	1510, $\Delta = -22\%$	1970(107%)
FEV_1/FVC	0.82	0.73	0.73
FEV_3/FVC	0.98		0.90
PFR (L/sec)	6.6		5.32
$FEF_{25-75\%}$	1.91(79%)		1.48(62%)
$FEF_{50\%}$	2.80		1.84
$FEF_{75\%}$	0.71		0.47
MVV (L/min)	82.3(124%)		80(127%)
D_LCO_{SB} (cc/min/Torr)	15.2(77%)		12.3(62%)
Hemoglobin gm/dl	14.2		10.5

*See footnote to Table 1-1, page 7, for description of predicted values used for Tables
showing pulmonary function test results.

receptors. The increase in reactivity may contribute to the development of airways
obstruction in smokers.

Barter and Campbell[44] related reactivity to methacholine, response to BD and
smoking to the rate of decline in FEV_1 in chronic bronchitis, using the post-BD
value for this measurement. Both indices of bronchial responsiveness correlated
with deterioration in ventilatory function. Progression of abnormality depended on
the interaction between reactivity and smoking. Even minimal smoking led to
serious deterioration when reactivity was high, whereas heavy smoking caused little
decrease in FEV_1 when reactivity was slight.

Dahms[45] demonstrated a 20 percent decrease in FVC, FEV_1, and flows in 10
asthmatics exposed to sidestream smoke. The tobacco smoke itself acted as a
provocational agent.

Bronchial irritants other than tobacco smoke induce or increase bronchial
reactivity. These include air pollutants like ozone and SO_2 and occupational irritants
and/or sensitizers like polyvinyl chloride pyrolysis products and dimethyl ethanol-
amine.

Selection of Patients for Treatment with Beta Blockers

Patients with CAO are at risk from bronchospasm if they are treated with beta blocking drugs. Cholinergic challenge identified the patients who later demonstrated deterioration with propranolol. A negative response indicates that patients are unlikely to develop bronchospasm.[46]

References

1. Hume KM, Gandevia B. Forced expiratory volume before and after isoprenaline. Thorax 12:276, 1957
2. Sourk RL, Nugent KM. Bronchodilator testing: Confidence intervals derived from placebo inhalations. Am Rev Respir Dis 128:153–157, 1983
3. Ramsdell JW, Tisi GM. Determination of bronchodilatation in the clinical pulmonary function laboratory: Role of changes in static lung volumes. Chest 76:622–628, 1979
4. Sherter CB, Connolly JJ, Schilder DP. The significance of volume-adjusting the maximal midexpiratory flow in assessing the response to a bronchodilator drug. Chest 73:568–571, 1978
5. Ries AL. Response to bronchodilators, in Clausen JL (Ed), Pulmonary function testing: Guidelines and controversies New York, Academic Press, 1982
6. Kanner, RE. The relationship between airways responsiveness and chronic airflow limitation. Chest 86:54–57, 1984
7. Committee on Emphysema, American College of Chest Physicians. Criteria for the assessment of reversibility in airways obstruction. Chest 65:552–553, 1974
8. Gross NJ, Skorodin MS. Anticholinergic, antimuscarinic bronchodilators. Am Rev Respir Dis 129:856–870, 1984
9. Dull WL, Alexander MR, Sadoul P, et al. The efficacy of isoproterenol inhalation for predicting the response to orally administered theophylline in chronic obstructive pulmonary disease. Am Rev Respir Dis 126:656–659, 1982
10. Mandella LA, Manfreda J, Warren CPW, et al. Steroid response in stable chronic obstructive pulmonary disease. Ann Intern Med 96:17–21, 1982
11. Ramsdell JW, Nachtwey FJ, Moser KM. Bronchial hyperreactivity in chronic obstructive bronchitis. Am Rev Respir Dis 126:829–832, 1982
12. Spector SL, Farr RS. A comparison of methacholine and histamine inhalations in asthmatics. J Allergy Clin Immunol 56:308–316, 1975
13. Juniper EF, Frith PA, Dunnett C, et al. Reproducibility and comparison of responses to inhaled histamine and methacholine. Thorax 33:705–710, 1978
14. Malo J, Pineau L, Cartier A, et al. Reference values of the provocative concentrations of methacholine that cause 6% and 20% changes in forced expiratory volume in one second in a normal population. Am Rev Respir Dis 128:8–11, 1983
15. Pepys J, Hutchcroft BJ. Bronchial provocation tests in etiologic diagnosis and analysis of asthma. Am Rev Respir Dis 112:829–859, 1975
16. Schoeffel RE, Anderson SD, Altounyan RE. Bronchial hyperreactivity in response to inhalation of ultrasonically nebulized solutions of distilled water and saline. Br Med J 283:1285–1287, 1981
17. Elwood RK, Hogg JC, Pare PD. Airway response to osmolar challenge in asthma. Am Rev Respir Dis (suppl) 125:61, 1982

18. Hogg JC, Eggleston PA. Is asthma an epithelial disease? (editorial) Am Rev Respir Dis 129:207–208, 1984

19. Mellis CM, Levison H. Bronchial reactivity in cystic fibrosis. Pediatrics 61:446–450, 1978

20. O'Byrne PM, Ryan G, Morris M, et al. Asthma induced by cold air and its relation to nonspecific bronchial responsiveness to methacholine. Am Rev Respir Dis 125:281–285, 1982

21. Deal EC Jr, McFadden ER Jr, Ingram RH Jr, et al. Airway responsiveness to cold air and hyperpnea in normal subjects and in those with hay fever and asthma. Am Rev Respir Dis 121:621–628, 1980

22. O'Cain CF, Dowling NB, Slutsky AS, et al. Airway effects of respiratory heat loss in normal subjects. J App Physiol Respirat Environ Ex 49:875–880, 1980

23. Anderson SD, Schoeffel RE, Daviskas E, et al. Exercise-induced asthma without airway cooling? Am Rev Respir Dis (suppl) 127:228, 1983

24. Phillips YY, Jaeger JJ, Laube BL, et al. Eucapanic voluntary hyperventilation of compressed gas mixture. A simple system for bronchial challenge by respiratory heat loss. Am Rev Respir Dis 131:31–35, 1985

25. Chai H, Farr RS, Froehlich LA, et al. Standardization of bronchial inhalation challenge procedures. J Allergy Clin Immunol 56:323–327, 1975

26. Corrao WM, Braman SS, Irwin RS. Chronic cough as the only presenting manifestation of bronchial asthma. N Engl J Med 300:633–637, 1979

27. Cockcroft DW, Killian DN, Mellon JJA, et al. Bronchial reactivity to inhaled histamine. A method and clinical survey. Clin Allergy 7:235–243, 1977

28. Cropp GJA (Chairman). Guidelines for bronchial inhalation challenges with pharmacologic and antigenic agents. Amer Thoracic Soc News 11–19, Spring 1980

29. Taylor WW, Ohman JL, Lowell FC. Immunotherapy in cat-induced asthma. J Allergy Clin Immunol 61:283–287, 1978

30. Chester EH, Schwartz HJ. Study session on occupational asthma. J Allergy Clin Immunol 64:665–671, 1979

31. Brooks SM. The evaluation of occupational airways disease in the laboratory and workplace. J Allergy Clin Immunol 70:56–66, 1982

32. Hargreave FE, Ryan G, Thomson NC, et al. Bronchial responsiveness to histamine or methacholine in asthma: Measurement of clinical significance. J Allergy Clin Immunol 68:347, 1981

33. Bahous J, Cartier A, Ouimet G, et al. Nonallergic bronchial hyperexcitability in chronic bronchitis. Am Rev Respir Dis 129:216–220, 1984

34. Yan K, Salome CM, Woolcock AJ. Prevalence and nature of bronchial hyperresponsiveness in subjects with chronic obstructive pulmonary disease. Am Rev Respir Dis 132:25–29, 1985

35. Bechtel JJ, Starr T III, Dantzker DR, et al. Airway hyperreactivity in patients with sarcoidosis. Am Rev Respir Dis 124:759–761, 1981

36. Milligan DWA, Levison H. Lung function in children following repair of tracheo-oesophageal fistula. J Pediatrics 95:24–27, 1979

37. Smyth JA, Tabachnick E, Duncan WJ, et al. Pulmonary function and bronchial hyperreactivity in long-term survivors of bronchopulmonary dysplasia. Pediatrics 68:336–340, 1981

38. Givan D, Scott P, Jeglum E, et al. Lung function and airway reactivity of children 3 to 10 years after foreign body aspiration. Am Rev Respir Dis (Suppl) 123:158, 1981

39. Laughlin J, Elgen H. Pulmonary function abnormalities in children following near drowning accidents. Am Rev Respir Dis (Suppl) 123:158, 1981
40. Malo JL, Filiatrault S, Martin RR. Bronchial hyperexcitability to inhaled methacholine in young asymptomatic smokers. Environ Occup Health 121:248, 1980
41. Gerrard JW, Cockcroft DW, Mink JT, et al. Increased nonspecific bronchial reactivity in cigarette smokers with normal lung function. Am Rev Respir Dis 122:577–587, 1980
42. Welty C, Weiss ST, Tager IB, et al. The relationship of airways responsiveness to cold air, cigarette smoking, and atopy to respiratory symptoms and pulmonary function in adults. Am Rev Respir Dis 130:198–203, 1984
43. Kabiraj MV, Simonsson BG, Groth S, et al. Bronchial reactivity, smoking and alpha-$_1$ antitrypsin. A population based study of middle aged men. Am Rev Respir Dis 126:864–869, 1982
44. Barter CE, Campbell AH. Relationship of constitutional factors and cigarette smoking to decrease in 1-second forced expiratory volume. Am Rev Respir Dis 113:305–314, 1976
45. Dahms TE, Bolin JF, Slavin RG. Passive smoking. Effects on bronchial asthma. Chest 80:530–534, 1981
46. Popio KA, Jackson DH, Utell MJ, et al. Inhalation challenge with carbachol and isoproterenol to predict bronchospastic response to propranalol in COPD. Chest 83:175–179, 1983

12

Pediatric Pulmonary Function Testing

Meyer Kattan

THE TESTS AVAILABLE AT VARIOUS AGES

Pulmonary function testing can serve as a helpful guide to the physician caring for the child with pulmonary disease. Measurement of *tidal volumes* and *flows* can be carried out in neonates and small infants during quiet breathing using a tightly

PULMONARY FUNCTION TESTS: A   ISBN 0-8089-1764-4   Copyright © 1987 by Grune & Stratton
GUIDE FOR THE STUDENT AND HOUSE OFFICER   All rights of reproduction in any form reserved.

fitting face mask attached to a pneumotachograph. *Thoracic gas volume* can be measured by a body plethysmograph and total respiratory resistance with a forced oscillation technique.[1,2] Some investigators have used the crying *vital capacity* as an index of lung volume in infants.[3]

Flow rates at FRC have been measured in children between the ages of 3 and 5 years using a *partial expiratory flow-volume maneuver* (Fig. 12-1).[4,5] The FRC is determined by recording a reproducible end expiratory point during tidal breathing. The child then inspires and blows out forcefully. This maneuver does not require the child to inspire to TLC or to exhale to RV. *Peak expiratory flow* can be measured reliably in most children at 5 years. By 7 years of age the pulmonary function tests used in children are the same as those used in adults.

LUNG GROWTH AND DEVELOPMENT

The lung is not fully developed at birth. By the 16th week of intrauterine life, all the nonrespiratory airways are present. Most respiratory airways appear between the 16th week of gestation and birth.

Alveolar development starts relatively late in the 7th month of intrauterine life. The alveoli, as they exist in the adult, do not begin to appear until about 8 weeks of age. In the newborn, the terminal bronchioles give rise to respiratory bronchioles, transitional ducts and terminal saccules. By 2 months of age, alveolar multiplication begins and continues to about 8 years of age. Alveolar size begins to increase only after the age of 5 years.

With the increase in alveolar number, the elastic fibers are still not mature. The distribution and concentration of elastic fibers do not reach adult values until adolescence. Thus, it is evident that the lung structures grow at different rates and at different times. This pattern has been termed dysanaptic.[6]

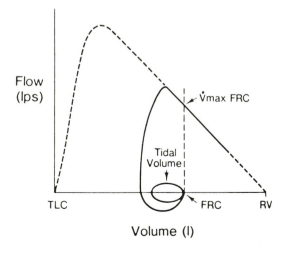

Fig. 12-1. Partial expiratory flow-volume curve (solid line). Maximal flow is measured at a reproducible FRC so that exhaling to RV is unnecessary. A full flow-volume curve is shown for comparison (dashed line). [From Taussig LM. Maximal expiratory flows at functional residual capacity: A test of lung function for young children. Am Rev Respir Dis 116:1032, 1977, with permission.]

There are several physiological consequences of these morphological features. Postnatally, the air exchange areas grow at a faster rate than the conducting system. Therefore, the lung volume to lung weight ratio and the alveolar volume-dead space ratio increase with age.[7,8] In the infant the lung elastic recoil pressure is lower, and airway closure occurs at end-expiration resulting in a lower arterial oxygen tension. Peripheral resistance is a large part of the total resistance until the age of 5 years. This is in contrast to the adult where resistance in the central airways has been thought to be the major part of total resistance.

Diffusion capacity is related to the surface area available for gas transfer. Therefore, as the lung grows, diffusion capacity increases. If the diffusion capacity is measured relative to lung volume, there is little change with age. However, in the neonatal period, diffusion capacity related to body surface area is approximately half the adult value.[9]

REPORTING RESULTS

Results of pulmonary function testing in children are as reproducible as they are in adults. In healthy children between the ages 7 and 16 years, the coefficient of variation of 6 to 8 repeated trials for FVC, FEV_1, PFR and $FEF_{50\%}$ are the same as in healthy young adults 17–18. Clinically, pulmonary function values can be used to distinguish "normal" from "abnormal" or to examine a patient's function over time. Identifying abnormal results requires a set of "normal" reference values. Several sets have been published.[10-13] Certain points, however, are noteworthy. In an adult, in whom only minor changes in body size occur with time, age is a major variable in determining pulmonary function. For evaluation of a child, age does not substantially influence the pulmonary function if height is used as the variable.[14]

In children, there is convincing evidence of differences in pulmonary function between males and females.[14-16] Blacks have lower values for lung volume and flow rates than Caucasians; this is thought to be in part due to the smaller sitting to standing height ratio in Blacks. Somewhat lower values in Mexican-Americans compared to Caucasians have also been demonstrated.[10] Regression equations based on height, sex and race are shown in Tables 12-1 and 12-2.

Data from a longitudinal study have provided standard values for the distribution of FVC and FEV_1 by height and sex for preadolescent (ages 6 to 11 years) white and black children.[14] The authors found that preadolescent children track along constant percentile curves of FVC and FEV_1. Therefore, one can monitor deterioration or improvement over time in an individual. Growth charts of pulmonary function are shown in Figures 12-2 and 12-3. Growth of lung function during adolescence differs from that of younger children; therefore, one cannot apply these curves to children above 11 years of age.

Table 12-1

Pediatric Regression Equations for Spirometry and Flows

		Males	Females
FVC*	Black	$1.07 \times 10^{-3} \times H^{2.93}$	$8.34 \times 10^{-4} \times H^{2.98}$
(L)	MA	$1.06 \times 10^{-3} \times H^{2.97}$	$1.25 \times 10^{-3} \times H^{2.92}$
	White	$3.58 \times 10^{-4} \times H^{3.18}$	$2.57 \times 10^{-3} \times H^{2.78}$
FEV_1*	Black	$1.03 \times 10^{-3} \times H^{2.92}$	$1.14 \times 10^{-3} \times H^{2.89}$
(L)	MA	$1.73 \times 10^{-3} \times H^{2.85}$	$1.61 \times 10^{-3} \times H^{2.85}$
	White	$7.74 \times 10^{-4} \times H^{3.00}$	$3.79 \times 10^{-3} \times H^{2.68}$
$FEF_{25-75\%}$	Black	$3.61 \times 10^{-4} \times H^{2.60}$	$1.45 \times 10^{-3} \times H^{2.34}$
(L/sec)	MA	$9.13 \times 10^{-4} \times H^{2.45}$	$1.20 \times 10^{-3} \times H^{2.40}$
	White	$7.98 \times 10^{-4} \times H^{2.46}$	$3.79 \times 10^{-3} \times H^{2.16}$
PFR†	Black	$2.26 \times 10^{-3} \times H^{2.39}$	$4.59 \times 10^{-3} \times H^{2.25}$
(L/sec)	MA	$8.21 \times 10^{-3} \times H^{2.15}$	$9.28 \times 10^{-3} \times H^{2.12}$
	White	$3.15 \times 10^{-3} \times H^{2.33}$	$1.63 \times 10^{-2} \times H^{2.00}$
$FEF_{50\%}$‡ (L/sec)		$Antilog_{10} (0.00795 \times H - 0.690)$	$Antilog_{10} (0.00894 \times H - 0.851)$
$FEF_{75\%}$‡ (L/sec)		$Antilog_{10} (0.00931 \times H - 1.252)$	$Antilog_{10} (0.00870 \times H - 1.128)$
MVV‡ (L/min)		$Antilog_{10} (0.00808 \times H + 0.748)$	$Antilog_{10} (0.00837 \times H + 0.690)$

*Hsu et al, 1979[10]
†Hsu et al, 1979[11]
‡Weng et al (1969 and unpublished data)[13]
H = height in cm, MA = Mexican Americans

Table 12-2

Pediatric Regression Equations for Static Lung Volumes

FRC		
(ml)	males	$1.10 \times 10^{-3} (H)^{2.84}$
	females	$4.52 \times 10^{-3} (H)^{2.55}$
RV		
(ml)	males and females	$1.17 \times 10^{-2} (H)^{2.22}$
TLC		
(ml)	males	$3.18 \times 10^{-3} (H)^{2.78}$
	females	$2.12 \times 10^{-3} (H)^{2.86}$

From Polgar C, Weng T-R. The functional development of the respiratory system: from the period of gestation to adulthood. Am Rev Respir Dis 120:625–695, 1979, with permission.
H = height in cm

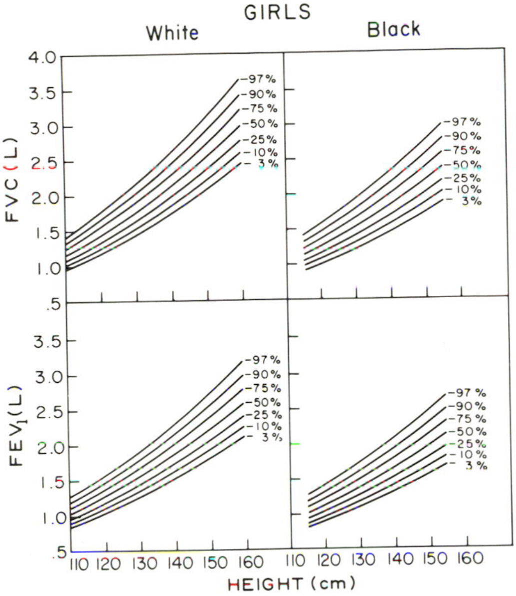

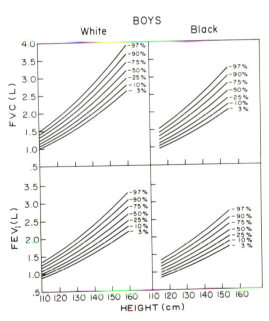

Fig. 12-2. Percentile curves of FVC and FEV₁ for white and black girls ages 6 to 11 years. [From Dockery DW, Berkey CS, Ware JH, et al. Distribution of forced vital capacity and forced expiratory volume in one second in children 6 to 11 years of age. Am Rev Respir Dis 128:410, 1983 with permission.]

Fig. 12-3. Percentile curves of FVC and FEV₁ for white and black boys ages 6 to 11 years [From Dockery DW, Berkey CS, Ware JH, et al. Distribution of forced vital capacity and forced expiratory volume in one second in children 6 to 11 years of age. Am Rev Respir Dis 128:411, 1983, with permission.]

ARTERIAL BLOOD GASES

These provide the most direct information regarding air exchange. Blood gases can be obtained at any age and are the most practical test under the age of 5. Lung development has a direct effect on the normal arterial oxygen values. Arterial oxygen increases in childhood, reaches a peak in the teenage years and declines thereafter (Fig. 12-4).[17] The lower oxygen value at young ages can be explained by the lower FRC. Airways may close at end expiration, resulting in greater mismatching of ventilation and perfusion.

"Arterialized" capillary blood samples reliably reflect arterial PO_2 in older children if careful technique is used.[18] They are not reliable in the first few days of life (they underestimate the arterial PO_2 when the true value is greater than 60 mm Hg); and in patients with impaired blood flow (eg, shock).

Transcutaneous PO_2 electrodes reflect trends in oxygenation and if calibrated can be a useful estimate of arterial PO_2.[19] Adequate circulation is necessary. For this reason, transcutaneous values cannot replace actual measurements of PO_2. Ear oximetry accurately measures oxygen saturation except at very low values.[20] However, the ears of younger children may be too thin to allow reliable recording.

AIRWAY FUNCTION

Airway Resistance

Airway resistance in children can be measured directly using a variable pressure body plethysmograph.[21] The panting maneuver required can be performed by most children over the age of 7 years.

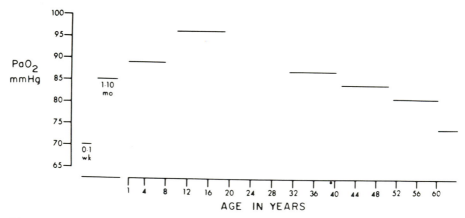

Fig. 12-4. Arterial oxygen tension at various ages. Values are lowest in infants and older adults. [From Bryan AC, Mansell AL, Levison H. Development of the mechanical properties of the respiratory system, in Hodson WA (Ed), Development of the lung. New York, Marcel Dekker 1977 p. 456, with permission.]

Peak Flow Rate

The PFR is simple to perform and yields reliable information in children by the age of five years. The subject is instructed to inspire to TLC and then to exhale as fast as possible; there is no need to exhale completely. The test is most useful in asthma.

Spirometry and Maximum Expiratory Flow-Volume Curves

Most children over 6 years of age can perform the forced expiratory maneuver (also see Chapter 2). After approximately 25 percent of the FVC is expired, maximum flow is dependent on the elastic properties of the lung and the airway resistance, and is not significantly altered by increased effort.

The shape of the MEFV curve varies with age as seen in Figure 12-5.[17,22] The curve of the adolescent (11–15 years) is similar to that of the young adult except at low lung volumes where an abrupt cessation of flow may be seen. This is because flow is limited by inability to overcome chest wall resistance. Young children have curves bending inward similar to those of older people. The similarity between childhood and old age is also seen in closing volume and could be explained by the lower static recoil pressure in these age groups.

Closing volume measurements made above the age of 6 show that this parameter decreases to a minimum in the late teens and then progressively increases with age[23] (Fig. 12-6).

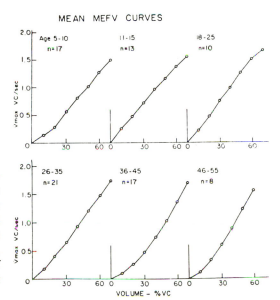

Fig. 12-5. Mean maximum expiratory flow-volume curves at various ages. The vertical axis represents flow in VC/sec and the horizontal axis volume as percent VC. See text for explanation. [From Green M, Mead J, Hoppin F, et al. Anaylsis of forced expiratory maneuver. Chest 63:345, 1973, with permission.]

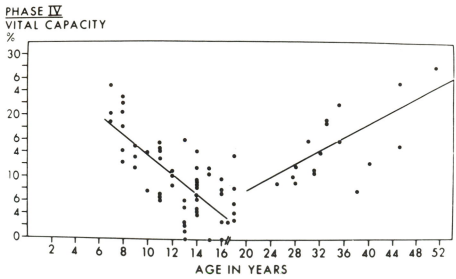

Fig. 12-6. Closing volume (Phase IV) expressed as percent of vital capacity as a function of age. The highest values are in young children and older adults. [From Mansell A, Bryan AC, Levison H. Airway closure in children. J Appl Physiol 33:712, 1972, with permission.]

EXERCISE TESTING

Children spend more time exercising than do adults. One can use exercise tests to estimate exercise tolerance (Chapter 15) or assess the degree of bronchial reactivity. Under the appropriate experimental conditions almost all children with asthma have evidence of airway obstruction following an exercise challenge.[24] However, in a routine pulmonary function laboratory where tests are done without prior conditioning of inspired air, exercise provocation is positive in 60–80 percent of asthmatics running on a treadmill.[25,26]

Children 6 years of age and over can run on a treadmill. Using a gradient of 10–15 percent, the speed is increased to achieve a heart rate 80–85 percent of the maximal (Fig. 12-7). This can be accomplished in less than 2 minutes. The duration of exercise is approximately 6 minutes at the suggested heart rate. Workload depends on the speed and slope of the treadmill, the subject's weight and pattern of exercise (eg, walking or running). Approximately 90 percent of asthmatic children can run for 6 minutes at the target exercise loads. In fact bronchodilatation is observed during the run. On the other hand, the remaining 10 percent of patients have severe bronchospasm within minutes of onset of exercise.

The usual pattern in asthmatics is airway obstruction that is maximal about 3–5 minutes after the cessation of exercise. The response to exercise challenge in normal and asthmatic children is shown in Figure 12-8. A fall in FEV_1 of more than 10

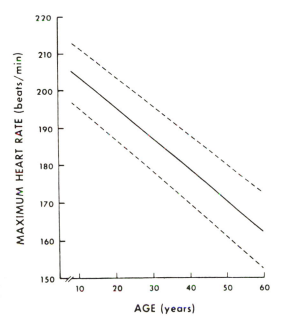

Fig. 12-7. Maximum predicted heart rate at various ages. The mean ± 1 SD are shown. [From Eggleston PA, Rosenthal RR, Anderson SA, et al. Guidelines for the methodology of exercise challenge testing of asthmatics. J Allergy Clin Immunol 64:644, 1979, with permission.]

percent or in PEF of more than 12.5 percent is considered a positive response.[25] It is generally unnecessary and unwise to exercise a patient for evidence of reactivity whose FEV_1 is less than 60 percent of predicted. In such cases it would be more informative to give a bronchodilator to determine reactivity.

PHARMACOLOGIC CHALLENGE

Human airways constrict when exposed to pharmacologic agents such as histamine and methacholine (see also Chapter 11). There is a spectrum of bronchoconstriction, normals being least sensitive to these agents and asthmatics most sensitive.

Fig. 12-8. The response to treadmill running in normal and asthmatic children. The bar represents the 6 minute period of running. The response is expressed as a percent of baseline peak flow rate. The data points are expressed as the mean ± SEM. [Adapted from data of Kattan M, Keens TG, Mellis CM, et al. The response to exercise in normal and asthmatic children. J Pediatr 92:718–721, 1978, with permission.]

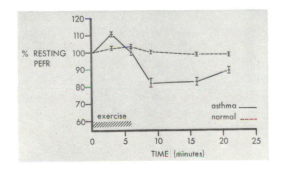

There are several advantages of pharmacologic challenge for determining bronchial reactivity. It can be used with a poorly coordinated child who has difficulty running on a treadmill or pedalling a bicycle. The response is more predictable and more easily controlled since the test is terminated after a 20 percent fall in FEV_1. This degree of reduction of airway function results in very little respiratory difficulty. Pharmacologic provocation is more sensitive in detecting airway reactivity in asthmatics than is the usual method of treadmill running.

CLINICAL APPLICATIONS OF PULMONARY FUNCTION TESTS

Asthma

Used dynamically, PFR is a simple and informative test. Once a baseline for a particular patient is determined, regular monitoring can serve to guide changes in medication. The test can be used in the home to document variations in airway function throughout the day. It can be used to establish responsiveness to a bronchodilator. Such information provides objective criteria for the physician before adding medications with potentially serious side effects to a treatment plan.

In asymptomatic children, the PFR and FEV_1 may be normal while flow rates at lower lung volumes are reduced.[27] The RV is usually increased. As obstruction becomes more severe, PFR and FEV_1 are reduced, RV is further increased with a reduction in FVC and specific airway conductance is decreased.

In children whose pulmonary function is normal the diagnosis of asthma may not be clear-cut. For example, cough as the primary manifestation of asthma can be difficult to distinguish from cough due to other causes. Therefore, one can take advantage of altered airway reactivity in asthma to establish the diagnosis.

Evaluation of Apnea

Obstructive apnea or hypopnea can be seen in children with hypertrophied tonsils and adenoids, hypopharyngeal collapse, and genetic disorders with macroglossia and/or micrognathia (see also Chapter 20). Apnea occurring in infants with "near miss" sudden infant death syndrome may be a result of lack of inspiratory effort (central apnea) or of upper airway obstruction.

Chest wall and abdominal excursion can be monitored by an impedance or inductance pneumograph (Respitrace). Air flow at the nose and mouth can be measured by thermistors or by a capnograph. Heart rate can be monitored with surface electrodes. Continuous monitoring of oxygenation can be achieved with an ear oximeter or transcutaneous oxygen electrode.

The predictive value of apnea monitoring in infants is less clear. Southall et al[28] prospectively recorded breathing in more than 9000 full term and premature infants. Of the 29 infants who had a sudden death, none had apneas greater than 20 seconds when studied. Moreover, none of the infants with prolonged apnea during the recording period died suddenly. Periodic breathing is usually defined as 3 respiratory pauses each of 3 or more seconds within a 20-second interval. Excessive periodic breathing or *short* "apneas" may be a risk factor for sudden death.[29]

Evaluation of Chronic Cough

Cough may be the sole manifestation of asthma. The diagnosis can be established readily if there is reversible airway obstruction. On the other hand, if pulmonary function is normal, bronchial provocation is helpful.

Cough may persist for months after upper respiratory tract infections. In pertussis, the paroxysmal cough can remain despite antibiotic treatment which eliminates the organism from the respiratory tract. Similarly cough may persist following a viral infection long after virus has disappeared. For 6 weeks following a viral illness, the airways may be hyperreactive to methacholine and histamine.[30] One explanation for the persistence of cough is that epithelial (cough) receptors have been sensitized.

In children and especially in adolescents, cough may be psychogenic (habit cough). The cough is usually harsh and barking and is extremely disturbing to those around the patient. A clue to the diagnosis is that while the cough is disruptive during the day, it does not occur while the patient is asleep. Pulmonary function is normal and bronchial hyperreactivity is absent.

Cystic Fibrosis

Cystic fibrosis is a genetic syndrome primarily affecting the exocrine glands. The diagnosis is established by elevated sweat electrolytes accompanied by one or more of the following features: chronic lung disease: pancreatic insufficiency: positive family history.

The earliest abnormalities in pulmonary function may be in small airway function.[31] Arterial oxygen tension is reduced because of mismatching of ventilation and perfusion. The RV and FRC are increased indicating air trapping. In older children with mild disease, the airway resistance and flows at high lung volumes may be normal because the peripheral resistance contributes a small proportion of the total resistance.

Progressive deterioration in expiratory flow rates and VC is demonstrated in the majority of patients. The RV and FRC increase further. The FEV_1/FVC decreases as the disease progresses, but the ratio may then rise as the FVC decreases more than the FEV_1.

With worsening disease, fibrotic changes occur in the lung, and a restrictive component is added to the obstructive disease. The TLC, as well as VC, are now reduced. The reduction in TLC magnifies the elevation in RV/TLC. Lung elastic recoil is little affected in the majority of patients.[32]

The PFR is not useful in cystic fibrosis. The bronchiectatic airways are more compliant. During a forced expiration, they are compressed, and the air contained in them is expelled early, contributing to the flows at high lung volume.[33]

Approximately 50 percent of patients with cystic fibrosis have evidence of bronchial hyperreactivity when challenged with methacholine.[34] The response to bronchodilator is variable.[35] It helps determine which patients may benefit from this treatment.

Scoliosis

Scoliosis is a deformity with both lateral curvature and rotation of the vertebrae. The most common pulmonary function abnormality is restriction of lung volumes.[36] The degree of curvature correlates with the reduction in lung volumes. In mild cases the pulmonary function is normal. In more severe cases there are reductions in TLC, VC, FRC, and compliance of the respiratory system. Residual volume may be normal, reduced or increased.[37,38] In general, the RV/TLC is elevated primarily because of a reduction in TLC. The FEV_1 and effort independent flow rates are normal if corrected for lung size.

Predicted lung function is based on height. One can use arm span to obtain the predicted values because arm span and expected height are similar. Gas exchange is affected in scoliosis. Arterial hypoxemia and an increased alveolar-arterial gradient for PO_2 are well documented.[39] The alveolar-arterial gradient, along with the dead space/tidal volume ratio, increase with age in patients with scoliosis. Maldistribution of ventilation and perfusion resulting from premature airway closure at end expiration has been observed.[40]

Patients who develop ventilatory restriction or in whom there is rapid progression of the angle of curvature require surgical correction. Immediately following surgery, there is a further reduction in lung volumes with restriction of chest movement because of pain and sedation.

Preoperative Evaluation of Pulmonary Function

Children with respiratory disease run a high risk of developing postoperative pulmonary complications. Postoperative respiratory failure is more than failure of the lungs; it may also be failure of the respiratory pump which includes the muscles and the chest wall. Some patients are able to cope with ventilatory requirements when well, but develop respiratory failure when complications develop.

It is necessary to determine whether there is adequate ventilatory capacity to cough and clear secretions. The average cough generates a flow of 4 to 6 L/sec. One needs an inspiratory capacity of approximately 15 cc/kg or a vital capacity about 40 percent of predicted to clear secretions. Therefore, in restrictive lung disease the risk of postoperative complications is increased as one approaches such values. Upper abdominal and thoracic operations result in the greatest decreases in VC, FRC and PFR. Godfrey found that if patients with scoliosis had a VC more than 40 percent of predicted, they did not have postoperative respiratory failure.[41]

References

1. Auld PAM, Nelson NM, Cherry RB, et al. Measurement of thoracic gas volume in the newborn infant. J Clin Invest 42:476–483, 1963
2. Doershuk CF, Downs TD, Matthews LW, et al. A method for ventilatory measurements in subjects one month to five years of age: Normal results and observations in disease. Pediatr Res 4:165–174, 1970
3. Sutherland JM, Ratcliff JW. Crying vital capacity. A simple and useful measure of lung volume in the newborn infant with respiratory disease. Am J Dis Child 101:67–74, 1961
4. Buist AS, Adams BE, Sexton GJ, et al. Reference values for functional residual capacity and maximal expiratory flow in young children. Am Rev Respir Dis 122:183–188, 1980
5. Taussig LM. Maximal expiratory flows at functional residual capacity: A test of lung function for young children. Am Rev Respir Dis 116:1031–1038, 1977
6. Green M, Mead J, Turner JM. Variability of maximum expiratory flow volume curves. J Appl Physiol 37:67–74, 1974
7. Mead J. Mechanical properties of the lung. Physiol Rev 41:281–330, 1961
8. Stigol LC, Vawter GF, Mead J. Studies on elastic recoil of the lung in a pediatric population. Am Rev Respir Dis 105:552–563, 1972
9. Krauss AN, Klain DB, Auld PAM. Carbon monoxide diffusing capacity in newborn infants. Pedatr Res 10:771–776, 1976
10. Hsu KHK, Jenkins DE, Hsi BP, et al. Ventilatory functions of normal children and young adults. Mexican, American, White and Black. I. Spirometry. J Pediatr 95:14–23, 1979
11. Hsu KHK, Jenkins DE, Hsi BP, et al. Ventilatory functions of normal children and young adults, Mexican, American, and Black. II. Wright peak flow meter and its use in pediatrics. J Pediatr 95:192–196, 1979
12. Polgar C, Promodhat V. Pulmonary function testing in children: Techniques and standards. Philadelphia, WB Saunders Company, 1971
13. Weng T-R, Levison H. Standards of pulmonary function in children. Am Rev Respir Dis 99:879–894, 1969
14. Dockery DW, Berkey CS, Ware JH, et al. Distribution of forced vital capacity and forced expiratory volume in one second in children 6 to 11 years of age. Am Rev Respir Dis 128:405–412, 1983
15. Dickman ML, Schmidt CD, Gardner RM. Spirometric standards for normal children and adolescents (ages 5 through 18 years). Am Rev Respir Dis 104:680–687, 1971
16. Zapletal A, Motoyama EK, Van de Woestiine KP, et al. Maximum expiratory flow-volume curves and airway conductance in children and adolescents. J Appl Physiol 26:308–315, 1969
17. Bryan AC, Mansell AL, Levison H. Development of the mechanical properties of the respiratory system, in Hodson WA (Ed), Development of the Lung. New York, Marcel Dekker, pp 455–468, 1977
18. Davis RH, Beran AV, Galant SP. Capillary pH and blood gas determinations in asthmatic children. J Allergy Clin Immunol 56:33–38, 1975
19. Huch R, Huch A, Albani M, et al. PO$_2$ monitoring in routine management of infants and children with cardiorespiratory problems. Pediatrics 57:681–690, 1976
20. Saunders NA, Powles ACP, Rebuck AS. Ear oximetry: Accuracy and practicability in the assessment of arterial oxygenation. Am Rev Respir Dis 113:745–749, 1976

21. Dubois AB, Botelho SY, Comroe JH Jr. A new method for measuring airway resistance in man using a body plethysmograph: values in normal subjects and patients with respiratory disease. J Clin Invest 35:327–335, 1956

22. Green M, Mead J, Hoppin F, et al. Analysis of forced expiratory maneuver. Chest 63:33S–35S, 1973

23. Mansell A, Bryan AC, Levison H. Airway closure in children. J Appl Physiol 33:711–714, 1972

24. Haynes RL, Ingram RH Jr, McFadden ER Jr. An assessment of the pulmonary response to exercise in asthma and an analysis of the factors influencing it. Am Rev Respir Dis 114:739–752, 1976

25. Kattan M, Keens TG, Mellis CM, et al. The response to exercise in normal and asthmatic children. J Pediatr 92:718–721, 1978

26. Shapiro GG, Pierson WE, Furukawa CT, et al. A comparison of the effectiveness of free running and treadmill exercise for assessing exercise-induced bronchospasm in clinical practice. J Allergy Clin Immunol 64:609–611, 1979

27. Weng T-R, Levison H. Pulmonary function in children with asthma at acute attack and symptom free status. Am Rev Respir Dis 99:719–728, 1969

28. Southall DP, Richards JM, de Sweet M, et al. Identification of infants destined to die unexpectedly during infancy: Evaluation of predictive importance of prolonged apnea and disorders of cardiac rhythm or conduction. Br Med J 286:1092–1096, 1983

29. Kelly DH, Shannon DC. Periodic breathing in infants with near-miss sudden infant death syndrome. Pediatrics 63:355–360, 1979

30. Empey DW, Laitinen LA, Jacobs L, et al. Mechanisms of bronchial hyperreactivity in normal subjects after upper respiratory tract infections. Am Rev Respir Dis 113:131–139, 1976

31. Mellins RB, Levine OR, Ingram RH Jr. et al. Obstructive disease of the airways in cystic fibrosis. Pediatrics 41:560–573, 1968

32. Mansell A, Dubrowsky H, Levison H, et al. Lung elastic recoil in cystic fibrosis. Am Rev Respir Dis 109:190–197, 1974

33. Landau LI, Taussig LM, Macklem PT, et al. Contribution of inhomogeneity of lung units to the maximum expiratory flow-volume curve in children with asthma and cystic fibrosis. Am Rev Respir Dis 111:725–731, 1975

34. Mitchell I, Corey M, Woenne R, et al. Bronchial hyper-reactivity in cystic fibrosis and asthma. J Pediatr 93:744–748, 1978

35. Kattan M, Mansell A, Levison H, et al. The response to aerosol salbutamol SCH 1000 and placebo in cystic fibrosis. Thorax 35:531–535, 1980

36. Weber B, Smith JP, Briscoe WA, et al. Pulmonary function in asymptomatic adolescents with idiopathic scoliosis. Am Rev Respir Dis 111:389–397, 1975

37. Kafer ER. Respiratory function in paralytic scoliosis. Am Rev Respir Dis 110:450–457, 1974

38. Kafer E. Respiratory and cardiovascular functions in scoliosis and the principles of anesthetic management. Anesthesiology 52:339–351, 1980

39. Kafer ER. Idiopathic scoliosis: Gas exchange and the age dependence of arterial blood gases. J Clin Invest 58:825–833, 1976

40. Bjure J, Grumby G, Gasalicky J, et al. Respiratory impairment and airway closure in patients with untreated idiopathic scoliosis. Thorax 25:451–456, 1970

41. Godfrey S. Respiratory and cardiovascular consequences of scoliosis. Respiration (suppl) 27:67–70, 1970

13

Surgical Considerations: Effects of Surgery on Lung Function; Preoperative Evaluation

Lee K. Brown

PULMONARY FUNCTION TESTS: A   ISBN 0-8089-1764-4   Copyright © 1987 by Grune & Stratton
GUIDE FOR THE STUDENT AND HOUSE OFFICER   All rights of reproduction in any form reserved.

A recent, comprehensive review of the effects of surgery on pulmonary function begins by quoting a fundamental precept of medicine, which dates back to the works of Hippocrates: *"primum non nocere"* ("first, do no harm").[1] This is a particularly apt beginning for a discussion of this type, for it is reasonable to expect a surgical procedure to improve the patient's status. However, a more modern quotation might be applied to this subject, "There is no such thing as a free lunch." That is to say, unavoidable changes in pulmonary function (both temporary and, in some cases, permanent) accompany many surgical procedures. It is the job of the clinician to anticipate these changes; to minimize them where possible, and to decide whether the surgery will do more harm than good.

EFFECTS OF SURGERY ON LUNG FUNCTION

Intubation, Mechanical Ventilation, and General Anesthesia

The profound intraoperative consequences of general anesthesia may be divided into effects on gas exchange, pulmonary mechanics and defense mechanisms.[2]

Gas Exchange—Oxygen

Oxygenation may be impaired by several mechanisms which cause ventilation-perfusion mismatching. First, progressive patchy atelectasis may occur during prolonged mechanical ventilation with low tidal volumes, presumably due to the preferential ventilation of lung units with the lowest resistance and highest compliance.[3] Earlier anesthesia practice included intermittent high volume breaths ("sighs"), which tended to prevent the atelectasis; current practice is to use high tidal volumes (10 ml/kg or more).[4,5] Second, the reduction in FRC that occurs in the supine and/or anesthetized subject,[6,7] especially if obese, leads to ventilation-perfusion mismatching if the FRC is below closing capacity (CC). Should this occur, dependent lung units will not be ventilated during part of each tidal breath.

Gas Exchange—CO₂

Decreases in CO_2 elimination have been widely reported during anesthesia. In patients still spontaneously ventilating, depressed central respiratory control may be partially implicated. Additionally in this group, and in those patients being mechanically ventilated, increases in dead space ventilation (V_D/V_T) occur.[8] This is primarily due to elevation of alveolar dead space caused by pulmonary hypotension with reduced perfusion of nondependent lung zones.[2,9,10]

Mechanics

The chest wall pressure-volume curve shifts to the right, and compliance increases, during mechanical ventilation, anesthesia, and muscle relaxation.[11] This shift was also seen when muscle relaxation was omitted;[12] volume history played a role, with higher tidal volumes resulting in more elevated compliance.

Lung pressure–volume relationships are altered in the opposite direction, with most studies demonstrating a reduction in C_L. This may be due to airway closure or patchy atelectasis, or changes in surfactant caused by mechanical ventilation or chemical effects of anesthetic gases.[2]

Pulmonary Defense Mechanisms

Coughing is considered the most effective process for clearance from the conducting airways; it involves a reflex neural pathway that may be blocked by a variety of anesthetic and narcotic agents. An effective cough also requires an intact glottis, which is obviously bypassed by intubation. Secondary defense mechanisms include phagocytosis of particles from the alveoli, transport of particles from alveoli to conducting system by surface forces of fluids, and transport of particles up the conducting airways by the mucociliary "escalator."[13] Intubation and/or anesthesia interferes with mucociliary transport. Anesthetic agents that have been shown to slow mucociliary transport include halothane,[14] ether,[15] and thiopental.[16]

Comment. While many of the changes associated with anesthesia and mechanical ventilation undoubtedly are reversed immediately after surgery, or are easily dealt with intraoperatively, it is likely that some linger into the postoperative period, especially if mechanical ventilation is continued. The alterations in defense mechanisms have great implications for the development of postoperative respiratory infections.

Abdominal and Nonresectional Thoracic Surgery

The changes in lung function occurring after abdominal or nonresectional thoracic surgery seem to be largely a consequence of incisional pain, the enforced supine postoperative position, and postoperative analgesia.

Lung Volumes

Presumably due to incisional pain limiting descent of the diaphragms (in abdominal surgery) and expansion of the chest (in thoracic surgery), VC decreases immediately following such procedures[17-20] while it remains unchanged following surgery elsewhere in the body.[18,19] In abdominal surgery, the decrease in VC varies with proximity of the incision to the diaphragms, high abdominal procedures having a greater effect. Beecher[17] and Anscombe[19] measured changes, which Wanner[21] has apparently used in an algorithm for preoperative screening (see below): VC (and presumably major timed volumes such as FEV_1) decreases about 50 percent following upper abdominal procedures, and 40 percent following lower abdominal surgery. In all studies, VC gradually returned toward normal over about two weeks' time. Changes in VC following major thoracic (nonresectional) surgery are similar in magnitude to those after high abdominal surgery.[20]

Anscombe[19] also studied static lung volumes, and subdivisions of VC, following abdominal surgery. The FRC decreases by about 20 percent following upper abdominal and 10% following lower abdominal surgery; the likely effect of this on gas exchange has already been discussed. The RV decreases slightly, if at all. The ERV decreases substantially (45 percent) in upper abdominal and less so (25 percent) in lower abdominal procedures. As ERV mainly represents diaphragmatic function, its sensitivity to upper abdominal procedures is not surprising.

Ventilatory Pattern

Minute ventilation is unchanged following laparotomy, but is achieved by using higher respiratory rates and lower tidal volumes.[17]

Gas Exchange

In the unintubated patient, the small tidal volumes and inhibition of the normal "sigh" may lead to progressive atelectasis and shunting. The reduction in FRC may lead to shunting if part of each tidal breath occurs below closing capacity. Additionally, V_D/V_T is increased as tidal volume is reduced.

Pulmonary Defense Mechanisms

Lack of effective cough due to postoperative pain, sedation, and the reduction in VC probably constitutes the most important abnormality. Additionally, ciliary function may be depressed as a residual effect of certain anesthetic agents (see above); and phagocytosis and clearing of bacteria may be inhibited by the hypoxemia which can occur postoperatively.[22]

Resectional Thoracic Surgery

In addition to the reversible changes in lung function following thoracotomy, resectional surgery results in permanent changes due to the removal of functional lung tissue. It should be pointed out that certain thoracic surgical procedures, both nonresectional and resectional, are performed in order to improve lung function. These include decortication, removal of bronchial obstruction (including sleeve resection and bronchoplasty, Case Presentation 13-1), resection of obstructed and/ or bronchiectatic lobes and resection of bullae.

Lung Volumes and Flows

Generally, VC and FEV_1 decrease in proportion to the amount of functional lung tissue resected. Thus, VC should be reduced by 55 percent following a right pneumonectomy and 45 percent following left pneumonectomy. For obvious reasons, the removed lung frequently was not normal functionally, and the actual decrease is usually less than predicted. The RV, FRC, and TLC are reduced approximately to the same extent as the VC.[23] Of note is the relatively minor reduction in MVV. This is not surprising, since lung resection amounts to an induced restrictive disorder, in which MVV may be spared by increasing respiratory rate (Chapter 4).

For less extensive resections, Juhl and Frost[24] have shown that the reduction in VC is about 300 cc less than 5.3 percent per segment removed. The FEV_1, FRC, and RV behaved similarly. The regression equation for FEV_1 was:

Equation 13-1

$$FEV_{1(post\ op.)} = 0.55 + 0.78\ X$$

where X is the preoperative FEV_1 reduced by 5.26 percent per segment resected.

Gas Exchange

Permanent changes following pulmonary resection are related to decreased surface area available for gas exchange and increased dead space.

Dietiker and coworkers[25] performed serial D_LCO_{SB} in 39 patients undergoing various surgical procedures. In those with resections, D_LCO_{SB} decreased in parallel with TLC, and D_LCO_{SB}/V_A remained unchanged, immediately post operatively. After a follow-up period of 4–21 months, D_LCO_{SB} increased while TLC remained the same. The increase in D_LCO_{SB}/V_A with time indicates a compensatory increase in gas transfer surface, possibly due to pulmonary capillary recruitment and increased blood flow.

Arterial blood gases at rest generally return to normal following resectional surgery, as does $P_{A-a}O_2$; the latter may increase on exercise, however.[26]

The V_D/V_T usually increases, probably reflecting both an increase in physiologic dead space and a decrease in tidal volume due to the restrictive defect of lung resection.[26,27] Distribution of ventilation, as assessed by multiple-breath N_2 washout, generally remains unchanged.[27,28]

Ventilatory Pattern and Control of Breathing

Respiratory rate increases and tidal volume decreases. However, respiratory drive as assessed by slope of $P_{0.1}$ response during CO_2 rebreathing remains unchanged.[29]

Hemodynamics

It is generally accepted that reduction of the pulmonary vascular bed by 50 percent in the normal individual (eg, by pneumonectomy) should not result in pulmonary hypertension. However, since pulmonary resection is frequently undertaken in patients with underlying lung disorders, a normal pulmonary vascular bed cannot be assumed. Thus, pulmonary hypertension is found in some patients following extensive resection; it may occur only during exercise.[28,30,31]

PREOPERATIVE EVALUATION

Indications

Indications for preoperative pulmonary function testing fall into two categories: *conditions* that are associated with increased risk of respiratory complications; and *procedures* that are associated with increased risk.

Not surprisingly, patients with any pulmonary disorder are at increased risk of atelectasis, pneumonia, bronchospasm, pulmonary embolus, and respiratory failure. Cigarette smoking, primarily because of its strong association with cardiopulmonary disease, is a known risk factor in surgery.

The association between postoperative morbidity and mortality and advanced age has been particularly well-studied. Burnett and McCaffrey,[33] for instance, evaluated the hospital course of 608 patients over the age of 70 who underwent major (mostly abdominal) procedures. Of these, 128 suffered pulmonary complications: bronchopneumonia (93), atelectasis (28), and pulmonary embolus (7). Preexisting lung disease, smoking, and immobility were associated risk factors.

Obesity, acting as a restrictive chest wall disorder, also increases the incidence of respiratory complications of surgery.[33,34]

Because of the profound changes in pulmonary function following upper abdominal or nonresectional thoracic surgery, preoperative evaluation is indicated when these procedures are anticipated.[17-19,35,38] Because these changes are reversible, this evaluation is largely a prediction of whether prolonged ventilatory support is likely to be required postoperatively.[37,38]

Prior to any contemplated lung resection, it is important to predict post-operative pulmonary function so that the patient does not end up a "pulmonary cripple."[23,39,40]

Finally, one should bear in mind that the preoperative testing should be done following suitable medical therapy for any preexisting pulmonary disorder to avoid counseling against surgery unnecessarily, and because postoperative outcome is improved.[41-43] Preoperative treatment decreased the incidence of pulmonary complications to near that of younger, "good risk" patients in one high risk series.[43]

Abdominal and Nonresectional Thoracic Surgery

One of the earliest quantitative approaches to preoperative screening was that of Miller, Wu and Johnson[44] (Table 13-1). Based on preoperative spirometry and postoperative clinical course in 24 patients, they developed an index based on the $FEV_{0.5}$ (expressed as percent FVC) and the percent predicted FVC:

Equation 13-2

$$k = \frac{\dfrac{FEV_{0.5}}{FVC} \times 100}{\dfrac{FVC}{Predicted\ FVC}} \times 100$$

This was useful in two respects: First, it separated patients into groups with obstructive, restrictive, combined obstructive/restrictive, and no impairment. Second, the value of k could be used in quantitating impairment, with a k below 0.15 constituting an extreme surgical risk.[45]

Table 13-1
Criteria for Assessing Postoperative Risk Based on Preoperative
Pulmonary Function Testing

Source	Parameter	Limits	Risk
Miller[45]	k (see Equation 13-2)	>0.5	Normal
		0.35–0.5	Mild
		0.25–0.35	Moderate
		0.15–0.25	Severe
		<0.15	Extreme
Peters[37]	$2.303 (FEF_{75-85\%})$	<3.387	Ventilatory
	$+ .0271 (P_E (max))$		support needed
Gracey[46]	MVV	<50% predicted	High
	+		probability
	$FEF_{25-75\%}$	<50% predicted	of complications
	+		
	FVC	<75% predicted	
Wanner[21]	Predicted	<10 L/M	Ventilatory
	$MSV_{post op.}$		support needed
	(see Equations 13-3 and 13-4)		

Peters[41] found that the combination of $FEF_{75-85\%}$ and maximal expiratory pressure ($P_E(max)$) correctly predicted the need for postoperative ventilatory support in 30 patients undergoing cardiac surgery (Table 13-1).

Gracey and coworkers[46] studied 157 patients with CAO. They concluded that patients with MVV and $FEF_{25-75\%}$ <50 percent of predicted and FVC <75 percent of predicted had a high probability of post-operative pulmonary complications (Table 13-1).

Finally, Wanner[21] has described a method, based on the FEV_1, that takes into account the type of surgery in a quantitative manner (Table 13-1). The MVV is calculated indirectly from the $FEV_1 \times 37.5$.

Since only about 60 percent of the MVV can be sustained indefinitely, an estimate of maximal sustained ventilation (MSV) is made:

Equation 13-3

$$MSV = 0.6 (37.5) (FEV_1)$$

Next, based on the data described above, the loss of FEV_1 due to the type of surgery is factored in:

Equation 13-4

$$MSV_{post op.} = (Fraction of FEV_1 remaining)(0.6) (37.5) (FEV_1)$$

Finally, a minimum postoperative minute ventilation of 10 L/m is assumed to be necessary to avoid respiratory complications. If the calculated $MSV_{post op.}$ is at or below this value, increased operative risk, and need for postoperative ventilatory support, is likely. For example, assume a preoperative FEV_1 of 0.8 L, and a planned upper abdominal procedure, leading to a 50 percent loss of FEV_1 immediately following surgery. Thus:

Equation 13-5

$$MSV_{post\ op.} = (0.5)\ (0.6)\ (37.5)\ (0.8) = 9\ L/M$$

Postoperative ventilatory support is deemed likely.

Resectional Thoracic Surgery

Gaensler et al[40] in one of the earliest studies using preoperative spirometry in lung surgery, evaluated 460 patients prior to thoracoplasty or resection for tuberculosis. The strong association between reduced MVV, reduced VC, and early respiratory failure set the stage for the current methods of screening candidates for lung resection.

Since pneumonectomy presents the greatest risk, methods predicting post-pneumonectomy ventilatory function are most numerous. In the bronchospirometric method[47,48] a Carlen's double-lumen endotracheal tube is introduced under topical anesthesia, and the VC, $\dot{V}_E$, and MVV of each lung measured individually, (The timed VC and oxygen consumption of each lung can be measured as well.) The postpneumonectomy VC is thus directly predicted.

Because bronchospirometry is invasive and not generally available, other techniques have been developed: radioisotopic ventilation or perfusion scanning, and the lateral position test.

As described by Miörner[49] and Kristersson and coworkers,[50,51] the portion of total ventilatory function attributable to each lung may be calculated by radioisotopic ventilation or perfusion scanning. The number of radioactive counts over each lung is divided by the total count to obtain the fractional contribution. This fractional contribution may then be multiplied by a preoperative measurement of function (eg. FEV_1) to predict remaining function after resection of the other lung. Using FEV_1, quantitative ventilation and perfusion scanning has been validated both against bronchospirometry[50] and against measured post-operative function.[24,50,52,53] Currently, [99m]Technetium perfusion scanning is most widely used because of the ease in obtaining and using the isotope (Fig. 13-1). Although FEV_1 is a measure of *ventilatory* function, local reflexes presumably match perfusion to ventilation well enough for a method based on regional *perfusion* alone to compare favorably to [133]Xenon ventilation scanning.[53]

An even less invasive method, the lateral position test (LPT), has also been used to predict post-pneumonectomy function. It is based on the observation that the increase in FRC that occurs in moving from the supine to the lateral decubitus position is proportional to the function of the uppermost lung (Fig. 13-2). While rebreathing a hyperoxic mixture from a spirometer (with CO_2 scrubber), the in-

Fig. 13-1. Postpneumonectomy FVC and FEV₁—actual versus predicted value using quantitative perfusion lung scanning. Straight line is that of identity. [From Olsen GN, Block AJ, Tobias JA. Prediction of postpneumonectomy pulmonary function using quantitative macroaggregate lung scanning. Chest 66:13, 1974, with permission.]

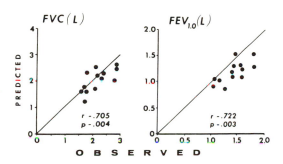

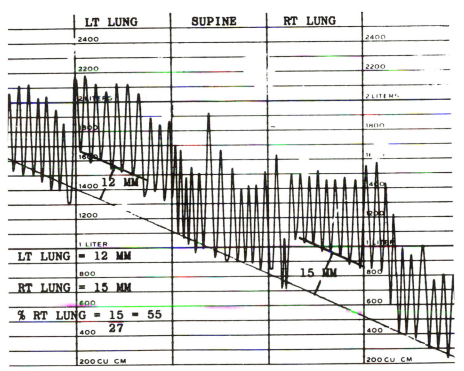

Fig. 13-2. Calculation of split pulmonary function using the lateral position test. Straight line defines FRC baseline (supine), which decreases with time due to O_2 consumption and CO_2 scrubbing from the closed system. Change in baseline (FRC) in moving to each lateral position is recorded, and split lung function calculated as shown. [From Marion JM, Alderson PO, Lefrak SS, et al. Unilateral lung function. Comparison of the lateral position test with radionuclide ventilation-perfusion studies. Chest 69:6, 1976, with permission.]

Table 13-3
Case Presentation 13-2

	10/4/83	10/25/83 (Post-bronchoplasty)	12/6/83 (stricture at bronchoplasty site)	4/24/84 (Post left pneumonectomy)
FVC (L)	2.12(52%)	2.87(71%)	2.94(74%)	1.86(47%)
FEV$_1$/FVC	0.72	0.70	0.59	0.74
FEV$_1$ (L)	1.52(53%)	2.01(71%)	1.73(62%)	1.38(50%)
MVV (L/min)	93.6 (91%)	103.2 (103%)	85(77%)	75.8 (73%)
Fraction of perfusion to right lung	—	0.63	0.73	—
Post-op FEV$_1$ (predicted from perfusion)	—	1.27 L	1.26	—
Fraction of ventilation to right lung	—	0.58	0.73	—
Post-op FEV$_1$ (predicted from ventilation)	—	1.17 L	1.26L	—

Note: Values in parenthesis are percent of predicted.

crease in FRC is measured separately between the supine and left and right lateral decubitus positions. These changes in FRC are summed. To calculate the contribution from the right lung, the increase in FRC from the supine to the left lateral decubitus position is divided by the sum of the FRC changes. This method has been validated against bronchospirometry, radioisotope scanning and post-operative pulmonary function, with some success,[54-59] but variability in test results is great. Quantitative scanning remains the preferred preoperative assessment.

The FEV_1 is the measurement usually chosen for prediction of postoperative function. This is primarily because epidemiologic data provide a specific value of FEV_1 (ie, 0.8 L) below which five-year mortality is prohibitive.[60] The FEV_1 also correlates quite well with MVV.

Most centers utilize recommendations similar to those of Block and Olsen:[61] clear patients for pneumonectomy if FEV_1 >2 L and >50 percent of FVC; MVV >50 percent predicted; RV/TLC <0.5. If all of these criteria are not met, clear for pneumonectomy if predicted postoperative FEV_1 is >0.8 L. If the latter criterion is not met, some centers would proceed to unilateral pulmonary artery occlusion, and clear for pneumonectomy if pulmonary hypertension is absent. Whether ventilatory function will be sufficient in these patients is unclear, however.

Smaller elderly subjects may not require an FEV_1 of 800 ml to sustain ventilation.

Case presentation 13-1 illustrates screening of the pneumonectomy candidate. A 63-year-old exsmoker presented with a five-month history of cough and wheezing. A localized wheeze was heard on the left. Standard PA and lateral chest radiographs were normal; an expiratory PA film showed hyperinflation on the left. Fiberoptic bronchoscopy revealed a mass partially obstructing the left main bronchus at the secondary carina. This was an intraepithelial squamous cell carcinoma on biopsy. Because of the "early" lesion, a sleeve resection and bronchoplasty were performed. Surgical margins were free of tumor. Postoperative studies showed improved pulmonary function, with FEV_1 increasing from 1.52 to 2.01 L (Table 13-3).

Over the ensuing two months, suture granulomas and fibrosis at the anastamosis caused recurrence of obstruction. Spirometry and quantitative lung scanning predicted a post-pneumonectomy FEV_1 of 1.26 L and a left pneumonectomy was performed. The FEV_1 several months following pneumonectomy was 1.38 L, in agreement with the predicted value. The patient was able to return to work.

References

1. Tisi GM. Preoperative evaluation of pulmonary function. Validity, indications and benefits. Am Rev Respir Dis 119:293–310, 1979
2. Rehder K, Sessler AD, Marsh HM. General anesthesia and the lung. Am Rev Respir Dis 112:541–563, 1975
3. Bendixen HH, Hedley-Whyte J, Laver MB. Impaired oxygenation in surgical patients during general anesthesia with controlled ventilation: A concept of atelectasis. N Engl J Med 269:991–996, 1963

4. Laver MB, Morgan J, Bendixen HH, et al. Lung volume, compliance, and arterial oxygen tensions during controlled ventilation. J Appl Physiol 19:725–733, 1964

5. Bendixen HH, Bullwinkel B, Hedley-Whyte J. et al. Atelectasis and shunting during spontaneous ventilation in anesthetized patients. Anesthesiology 25:297–301, 1964

6. Hewlett AM, Hulands GH, Nunn JF, et al. Functional residual capacity during anaesthesia. II. Spontaneous respiration. Br J Anaesth 46:486–494, 1974

7. Hewlett AM, Hulands GH. Nunn JF, et al. Functional residual capacity during anaesthesia. III. Artificial ventilation. Br J Anaesth 46:495–503, 1974

8. Campbell EJM, Nunn JF, Peckett BW. A comparison of artificial ventilation and spontaneous respiration with particular reference to ventilation-bloodflow relationships. Br J Anaesth 30:166–175, 1958

9. Askrog V. Changes in (a-A) CO_2 difference and pulmonary artery pressure in anesthetized man. J Appl Physiol 21:1299–1305, 1966

10. Nunn JF, Campbell EJM, Peckett BW. Anatomical subdivisions of the volume of respiratory dead space and effect of position of the jaw. J Appl Physiol 14:174–176, 1959

11. Westbrook PR, Stubbs SE, Sessler AD, et al. Effects of anesthesia and muscle paralysis on respiratory mechanics in normal man. J Appl Physiol 34:81–86, 1973

12. Grimby G, Hedenstierna G, Lofstrom B. Chest wall mechanics during artificial ventilation. J Appl Physiol 38:576–580, 1975

13. Kilburn KH. A hypothesis for pulmonary clearance and its implications. Am Rev Respir Dis 98:449–463, 1968

14. Forbes AR. Halothane depresses mucociliary flow in the trachea. Anesthesiology 45:59–63, 1976

15. Forbes AR, Gamsu G. Mucociliary clearance in the canine lung during and after general anesthesia. Anesthesiology 50:26–29, 1979

16. Forbes AR, Gamsu G. Thiopental depresses lung mucociliary clearance to the same extent as halothane. Abstracts of Scientific Papers, American Society of Anesthesiologists Annual Meeting. Chicago, 1978

17. Beecher HK. The measured effect of laparotomy on the respiration. J Clin Invest 12:639–650, 1933

18. Churchill ED, McNeil D. The reduction in vital capacity following operation. Surg Gynec Obst 44:483–488, 1927

19. Anscombe AR, Buxton R StJ. Effect of abdominal operations on total lung capacity and its subdivisions. Br Med J 2:84–87, 1958

20. Howatt WF, Talner NS, Sloan H, et al. Pulmonary function changes following repair of heart lesions with the aid of extracorporeal circulation. J Thoracic and Cardiovasc Surg 43:649–657, 1962

21. Wanner A. Interpretation of pulmonary function tests, in Sackner MA (ed), Diagnostic Techniques in Pulmonary Disease. New York, Marcel Dekker, 1980, pp 353–426

22. Harris GD, Johanson WG Jr, Pierce AK. Bacterial lung clearance in hypoxic mice. Am Rev Respir Dis 111:910, 1975

23. Boushy SF, Billig DM, North LB, et al. Clinical course related to preoperative and postoperative pulmonary function in patients with bronchogenic carcinoma. Chest 59:383–391, 1971

24. Juhl B, Frost N. A comparison between measured and calculated changes in the lung function after operation for pulmonary cancer. Acta Anaesth Scand 57 (suppl):39–45, 1975

25. Dietiker F, Lester W, Burrows B. The effects of thoracic surgery on the pulmonary diffusing capacity. Am Rev Respir Dis 81:830–838, 1960

26. Birath G, Malmberg R, Simonsson BG. Lung function after pneumonectomy in man. Clin Sci 29:59–72, 1965

27. Jones JC, Robinson JL, Meyer BW, et al. Primary carcinoma of the lung. A follow-up study including pulmonary function studies of long-term survivors. J Thoracic and Cardiovasc Surg 39:144–158, 1960

28. Burrows B, Harrison RW, Adams WE, et al. The postpneumonectomy state. Clinical and physiologic observations in thirty-six cases. Am J Med 28:281–297, 1960

29. Easton PA, Arnup ME, de la Rocha A, et al. Ventilatory control after pulmonary resection. Am Rev Respir Dis 128:627–630, 1983

30. Fry WA, Harrison RW, Moulder PV, et al. Serial study of postpneumonectomy state. Arch Surg 85:578–586, 1962

31. Cournand A, Riley RL, Himmelstein A, et al. Pulmonary circulation and alveolar ventilation-perfusion relationships after pneumonectomy. J Thoracic Surg 19:80–116, 1950

32. Gass GD, Olsen GN. Preoperative pulmonary function testing to predict postoperative morbidity and mortality. Chest 89:127–135, 1986

33. Burnett W, McCaffrey J. Surgical procedures in the elderly. Surg Gynec Obst 134:221–226, 1972

34. Gould AB. Effect of obesity on respiratory complications following general anesthesia. Anesth and Analg 41:448–452, 1962

35. Putnam L, Jenicek JA, Allen CR, et al. Anesthesia in the morbidly obese patient. South Med J 67:1411–1417, 1974

36. Stein M, Koota GM, Simon M, et al. Pulmonary evaluation of surgical patients. JAMA 181:765–770, 1962

37. Miller RD. Evaluation of pulmonary impairment in the surgical candidate. Med Clin North Am 46:885–890, 1962

38. Peters RM, Brimm JE, Utley JR. Predicting the need for prolonged ventilatory support in adult cardiac patients. J Thoracic and Cardiovasc Surg 77:175–182, 1979

39. Redding JS, Yakaitis RW. Predicting the need for ventilatory assistance. Maryland State Med J 19:53–57, 1970

40. Mittman C. Assessment of operative risk in thoracic surgery. Am Rev Respir Dis 84:197–207, 1961

41. Gaensler EA, Cugell DW, Lindgren I, et al. The role of pulmonary insufficiency in mortality and invalidism following surgery for pulmonary tuberculosis. J Thorac Surg 29:163–187, 1955

42. Hodgkin JE, Dines DE, Didier EP. Preoperative evaluation of the patient with pulmonary disease. Mayo Clin Proc 48:114–118, 1973

43. Miller WF, Cade JR, Cushing IE. Preoperative recognition and treatment of bronchopulmonary disease. Anesthesiology 18:483–497, 1957

44. Stein M, Cassara EL. Preoperative pulmonary evaluation and therapy for surgery patients. JAMA 211:787–790, 1970

45. Miller WF, Wu N, Johnson RL Jr. Convenient method of evaluating pulmonary ventilatory function with a single breath test. Anesthesiology 17:480–493, 1956

46. Miller WF. Preoperative evaluation of pulmonary function in the surgical patient, in Chusid EL (Ed), The Selective and Comprehensive Testing of Adult Pulmonary Function. Mt. Kisco. NY, Futura, 1983, pp 283–296

47. Gracey DR, Divertie MB, Didier EP. Preoperative pulmonary preparation of patients with chronic obstructive pulmonary disease. Chest 76:123–129, 1979

48. Snider GL. A critical evaluation of bronchospirometric measurement in predicting loss of ventilatory function due to thoracic surgery. J Lab Clin Med 64:321–329, 1964

49. Neuhaus H, Cherniack NS. A bronchospirometric method of estimating the effect of pneumonectomy on the maximum breathing capacity. J Thoracic Cardiovasc Surg 55:144–148, 1968

50. Miörner G. ^{133}Xe-radiospirometry. A clinical method for studying regional lung function. Scand J Resp Dis 64 (suppl), 1968

51. Kristersson S, Lindell S-E, Svanberg L. Prediction of pulmonary function loss due to pneumonectomy using ^{133}Xe-radiospirometry. Chest 62:694–698, 1972

52. Kristersson S, Arborelius M Jr, Jungquist G, et al. Prediction of ventilatory capacity after lobectomy. Scand J Resp Dis 54:315–325, 1973

53. Olsen GN, Block AJ, Tobias JA. Prediction of postpneumonectomy pulmonary function using quantitative macroaggregate lung scanning. Chest 66:13–16, 1974

54. Boysen PG, Block AJ, Olsen GN, et al. Prospective evaluation for pneumonectomy using the ^{99m}Technetium quantitative perfusion lung scan. Chest 72:422–425, 1977

55. Bergan F. The relative function of the lungs in supine, left and right lateral positions. J Oslo City Hosp 2:185–197, 1952

56. Bergan F. A simple method for the determination of the relative function of the right and left lung. Acta Chir Scand 253 (suppl):58–63, 1960

57. Hazlett DR, Watson RL. Lateral position test: A simple, inexpensive, yet accurate method of studying the separate functions of the lungs. Chest 59:276–279, 1971

58. DeMeester TR, Van Heertum RL, Karas JR, et al. Preoperative evaluation with differential pulmonary function. Ann Thorac Surg 18:61–71, 1974

59. Marion JM, Alderson PO, Lefrak SS, et al. Unilateral lung function. Comparison of the lateral position test with radionuclide ventilation-perfusion studies. Chest 69:5–9, 1976

60. Walkup RH, Vossel LF, Griffin JP, et al. Prediction of postoperative pulmonary function with the lateral position test. Chest 77:24–27, 1980

61. Diener CF, Burrows B. Further observations on the course and prognosis of chronic obstructive lung disease. Am Rev Respir Dis 111:719–724, 1975

62. Block AJ, Olsen GN. Preoperative pulmonary function testing. JAMA 235:257–258, 1976

14

Assessment of Respiratory Impairment and Disability

Albert Miller
David J. Kanarek

PULMONARY FUNCTION TESTS: A   ISBN 0-8089-1764-4   Copyright © 1987 by Grune & Stratton
GUIDE FOR THE STUDENT AND HOUSE OFFICER   All rights of reproduction in any form reserved.

Pulmonary Function Evaluation
  Noninvasive Tests
    Spirometry
    Diffusing Capacity
    Lung Volumes
  Arterial Blood Gases
Schemes for Evaluating Respiratory Impairment
  American Thoracic Society
  Social Security Administration
  American Medical Association
Integration of Clinical and Laboratory Findings

DEFINITIONS

Impairment has been defined as the loss of function.[1] The American Thoracic Society[2] states that impairment "reflects a functional abnormality that persists after appropriate therapy and with no reasonable prospect of improvement." The 1984 American Medical Association *Guides to the Evaluation of Permanent Impairment* defines impairment as an alteration of health status defined by medical means.[3]

It is the responsibility of the physician to quantitate the impairment and to draw conclusions about the individual's physical capacity. Clinical evaluation complemented by resting pulmonary function studies may provide adequate information. If these are insufficient, exercise studies may be utilized.

In contrast, *disability* is defined as the inability to perform at a specified level of activity[4] or as undue distress during the performance of that task.[5] The 1984 AMA Guides defines disability as an alteration of the capacity to meet personal, social or occupational demands, or to meet statutory or regulatory requirements.[3] The earlier AMA guidelines[6] referred to a "reduction or absence of ability to engage in gainful activity . . . because of impairment." It is obvious that determination of disability is a complex administrative decision that includes impairment among a number of factors such as education, training, experience, the requirements of a job, age, and motivation. The physician's input is important but is only part of the process. Disability may be complete or partial, permanent or temporary.

The physician's conclusion must include the diagnoses, the contributing factors, the nature and extent of physiologic impairment, and, where requested, the influence of the impairment on the ability to carry out specific tasks. This Chapter will deal most extensively with the last two elements.

MEDICAL HISTORY

Occupational History

This should describe accurately all the jobs in chronological sequence, together with the duration, contact with known toxic materials, protective devices and any other specific hazards.

Smoking

Cough and Sputum Production

Frequent coughing, copious sputum production, or hemoptysis may make it difficult to carry out a task properly, such as delicate hand work or dealing with the public (eg, as a receptionist).

Wheezing

The timing of wheezing in relation to work hours, the duration of the episodes and the presence of atopy are helpful in separating asthma of occupational origin.

Chest Pain

This may cause disability by itself.

DYSPNEA

Definition

Dyspnea is by far the most important symptom causing disability of pulmonary origin. Dyspnea is an *awareness* of the effort of breathing; effort can be thought of as the efferent drive from the central nervous system to the inspiratory muscles. It involves the processing of sensory information converging on integrating centers in the brain both from the respiratory apparatus and from elsewhere in the body (Table 14-1). It also involves the interpretation of these sensations. Lay terms are "shortness of breath" or "breathlessness" (to be distinguished from the "inability to take a deep breath" of the patient with anxiety or hyperventilation syndrome, often described to the physician in great length and with little pause).

Dyspnea may therefore be normal or abnormal. Dyspnea during exercise is abnormal when it is perceived at a level of exertion that is ordinarily tolerated without awareness of undue effort. Dyspnea may serve a beneficial purpose by limiting the work of breathing and thus forestalling fatigue of the respiratory muscles and further respiratory failure.

Table 14-1
Neural Pathways for Dyspnea

Receptors
    Lung—irritant, ? stretch (vagal); information about change in
        lung volume and transpulmonary pressure.
    Lung—"J" (alveolar septa): information about circulation
    Chest Wall—muscle spindles may sense appropriateness of
        tension (developed in inspiratory muscles by CNS drive) and
        length of the fibers (volume of the breath achieved)
    Atrial—stretch
    Skeletal muscles elsewhere in body
    Chemo (O_2, CO_2, pH)
Integrating center in brain (reticular activating system)

Correlates on Physical Examination

Certain findings on physical examination are considered evidence of dyspnea, eg, pursed lips breathing or inability to complete a sentence.[3] Mohler[7] lists the following 10 signs: length of word string, stress quality of voice, mouth breathing, use of accessory muscles, supraclavicular retraction, intercostal retraction, head rocking, fish mouth breathing, flaring of alae nasae, and pupillary dilatation.

Physiologic Correlates

Dyspnea secondary to pulmonary disease can generally be explained by increases in ventilation and work of breathing, and/or by decrease in respiratory muscle strength.

Increased Minute Ventilation ($\dot{V}_E$)

Increased V_D/V_T is a major contributor to increased $\dot{V}_E$ in lung disease. Stimulation of chemoreceptors by hypoxemia or acidosis increases $\dot{V}_E$; exercise-associated fall in PaO_2 is characteristic of ILD and emphysema. The breathing reserve ratio relates actual ventilation ($\dot{V}_E$) to the capacity for ventilation, measured by the MVV:

Equation 14-1

$$\text{Breathing reserve ratio} = \frac{MVV - \dot{V}_E}{MVV} \times 100$$

A value less than 60 is associated with dyspnea. eg, *Normal* subject, moderate exercise:

$$\frac{160 - 40}{160} \times 100 = 75 \text{ (no dyspnea)}$$

Patient with *severe CAO*, rest:

$$\frac{25 - 12.5}{25} \times 100 = 50 \text{ (severe dyspnea)}$$

Increased Work of Breathing Against Elastic or Frictional Forces

Respiratory patterns.   These patterns achieve the least work against elastic forces by decreasing tidal volume and increasing rate. Although the respirations in patients with airway obstruction should be deep and slow in order to minimize work against frictional resistance, these patients are seen to breathe rapidly and shallowly. This is because the increase in FRC secondary to air trapping shifts the volume-pressure curve to its flatter portion close to TLC. The physiologic trade-off is that bronchial diameter is increased, lessening work against resistive forces.

A consequence of rapid shallow breathing (in ILD and in airways obstruction) is decreased tidal volumes and increased V_D/V_T.

Inspiratory flow.   Dyspnea is generated primarily during *inspiration*. The mechanism for dyspnea when airway resistance is increased on *expiration* is limitation in the time available for inspiration, thus requiring an increase in inspiratory flow. Mean inspiratory flow, or tidal volume/inspiratory time (V_T/T_I), is used as an index of *respiratory drive*. Dyspnea has been related to this measurement when it is expressed as a percentage of the maximum inspiratory flow (easily measured as part of the maximum inspiratory flow-volume curve). Dyspnea was perceived at 15 percent of the maximum inspiratory flow and increased linearly in magnitude, reaching the fatigue level at 40 percent.[8] This index, $\dot{V}_{insp}$ % max, quantitatively reflects the proportion of inspiratory muscle capacity utilized and is influenced both by the tension generated by the respiratory muscles and by their strength.

In upper airways obstruction, peribronchial fibrosis, and to some extent chronic bronchitis, airway resistance is increased on inspiration, heightening the load on inspiration, and the sensation of dyspnea.

Respiratory muscle fatigue.   Hypoxia and lactic acidosis of the respiratory muscles contribute to their fatigue. This is the major reversible element when respiratory failure supervenes in restrictive impairments of the chest cage.

Correlation with pulmonary function tests.   Since elastic and resistive forces can be measured by simple pulmonary function tests, the former by VC and the latter by FEV_1, R_{aw}, and flows, these may be expected to show a good correlation with dyspnea when dyspnea is *due to* abnormal mechanical forces.

Decreased Strength of the Respiratory Muscles

This is measured as the maximum pressures generated at the mouth, P_{Imax} (measured at RV or FRC) and P_{Emax} (measured at TLC). These measurements are markedly reduced in neuromuscular disease (see Chapter 10) but are reduced in lung disease as well, both because of alterations in the length : velocity relationship as diaphragmatic curvature is reduced secondary to hyperinflation and because of associated muscle atrophy.

Length: Tension Inappropriateness

The classic concept that "explains" dyspnea, formulated by Campbell,[9] relates the tidal volume or minute ventilation achieved ("length") to the inspiratory neuromuscular drive that brought it about ("tension"): "For the amount of tension developed in the inspiratory muscles, the expansion of the chest is less than expected."

Cardiac Dyspnea

Dyspnea secondary to cardiac disease does not correlate well with changes in mechanical forces in the lungs in the absence of overt congestive heart failure. Both systolic (inotropic or contraction) and/or diastolic (lusitropic or relaxation) dysfunction of the heart may cause increased left ventricular and therefore pulmonary capillary pressure and reduced pulmonary compliance. Dyspnea may result from impaired ventricular relaxation (reduced myocardial compliance) even when the ejection fraction is well maintained. In this situation, heart size is often normal.

Hyperventilation, especially on exercise with an early onset of anaerobic threshold, and muscle weakness are likely to be present in patients with heart disease. Decreased cardiac output and pulmonary perfusion, and pulmonary hypertension probably play roles in causing dyspnea.

Grading

Dyspnea is subjective and difficult to quantify precisely. One grading system, based on the British Medical Research Council questionnaire (shown in Table 14-2), requires from the subject some perception of how others perform. Grade 1 on this scale is normal. Dyspnea correlates with increasing pulmonary impairment.[10,11] However, the scatter is wide and, in a particular individual, the FEV_1 cannot be predicted from the severity of the complaint.

Table 14-2
Grading of Dyspnea

Grade I	Dyspnea on vigorous effort only.
Grade II	Troubled by inclines or when hurrying on level ground.
Grade III	Short of breath walking with others of similar age and physique, even on level ground, but can walk a mile slowly, do own shopping.
Grade IV	Short of breath with mild activities; cannot walk one block or climb one flight of stairs without stopping for breath.

Modified from Medical Research Council, Committee on the Aetiology of Chronic Bronchitis. Standardized questionnaires on respiratory symptoms. Br Med J 2:1665, 1960

PHYSICAL EXAMINATION

The physical examination, while lacking sensitivity, permits a broad assessment of the type and degree of pulmonary impairment. Prolonged forced expiration, wheezing, distant breath sounds, and crackles are helpful in obstructive or interstitial disease. Second, it suggests other primary or contributory causes of dyspnea such as obesity, cyanosis, plethora, cardiac disorders, and pulmonary hypertension.

CHEST X-RAY

Radiographs are important in diagnosis but have a poor correlation with the degree of pulmonary impairment unless the impairment is severe. Late stages of CAO *may* show hyperinflation, and restrictive pulmonary impairment is generally accompanied by an interstitial infiltrate.

PULMONARY FUNCTION EVALUATION

Pulmonary function tests are the mainstay of impairment evaluation and are used to classify impairment by grade of severity (Tables 9-1–9-6) and by physiologic categories (Chapter 10). Tests provide objective evidence of impairment. Particularly when impairment is severe, results can be related to dyspnea.

Noninvasive tests

Spirometry

The VC and FEV_1 are the basic tests. Severe deficits are evidence of sufficient disease to impair function. However, it must be noted that these are not tests of exercise capacity and that it is not possible to predict an individual's exercise performance from her FEV_1 or her VC, although a correlation exists when a large number of subjects are studied (Fig. 14-1) and low values must result in ventilatory limitation.

Diffusing Capacity

The D_LCO_{SB} is useful in assessing pulmonary vascular disorders and parenchymal destruction in ILD and in emphysema. It is the next test when spirometry does not indicate severe impairment.

Lung Volumes

The TLC is useful in defining restriction. The FRC and RV quantitate the degree of air trapping and help in understanding the significance of a reduced FVC. In evaluating disability, they add little to spirometry.

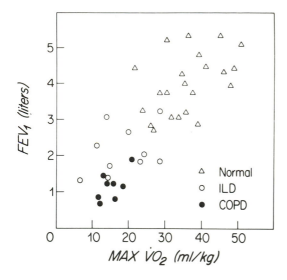

Fig. 14-1. The relationship between exercise capacity and FEV_1 in
normal subjects and in patients with
various lung diseases. Note relationship between FEV_1 and $\dot{V}O_{2max}$
achieved.

Arterial Blood Gases

These are discussed in Chapter 8 and in Chapter 15.

SCHEMES FOR EVALUATING RESPIRATORY IMPAIRMENT

Most schemes for evaluating respiratory impairment are based on resting pulmonary function tests. These test results are not assessed according to the subject's
occupational demands; a FVC of 2.5 L or 50 percent of predicted is the same degree
of impairment for an accountant as for a stevedore. The American Thoracic Society[2]
and the American Medical Association[3] include exercise criteria (see Chapter 15).

Clinicians equate total disability with severe impairment of FVC, FEV_1, and/or
MVV, and D_LCO. In addition, CO_2 retention, severe hypoxemia or clinical findings
such as secondary erythrocytosis, or evidence of pulmonary hypertension and cor
pulmonale may be accepted as proof of disability.

American Thoracic Society

The 1982[2] "official" guideline defined "severe impairment" as $FEV_1 \leq 40$
percent of predicted, FVC ≤ 50 percent of predicted, $FEV_1/FVC \leq 40$ percent of
predicted, and/or $D_LCO \leq 40$ percent of predicted. If pulmonary function results
are above these values in a dyspneic subject exercise testing was recommended (see
below). The 1986[12] statement revised the FEV_1/FVC criterion for severe impairment to ≤ 0.40 and added categories for mild and moderate impairment using
standard pulmonary function tests and $\dot{V}O_2$ max.

Social Security Administration

The Administration[13] adjudicates and awards compensation for total disability defined as the

> inability to engage in any substantial gainful activity by reason of a medically determinable physical or mental impairment which can be expected to result in death or that has lasted or can be expected to last for a continuous period of not less than 12 calendar months. . . . Impairment must be established by medical evidence consisting of signs, symptoms and laboratory findings.

Disability is based on "functional residual capacity" to meet occupational demands, which are classified as sedentary, light, medium, heavy, and very heavy. (Note that this is *not* the pulmonologist's *functional residual capacity!*)

The Social Security Handbook for Physicians[12] provides tables for assessing total respiratory impairment, using observed values adjusted for height, rather than percentage of predicted. The range of FEV_1 is 1.1 (height 60 inches) to 1.4 L (height 73 inches), of MVV 35–48 L/min, of VC (ILD) 1.4–2.0 L, and of VC (chest bellows disorder or resection of lung) 1.1–1.4 L. Since pulmonary function declines with age (and is lower in females and blacks), younger (male or Caucasian) claimants must experience a greater loss of function than older individuals to receive an award.

Criteria also include $D_L CO_{SB}$ < 30 percent of predicted (*which* predicted is not specified) or < 9 ml/min/mm Hg and low PaO_2 relative to $PaCO_2$ (≤ 56 mm Hg when $PaCO_2$ and pH are normal). For asthma, the frequency of severe episodes determines the level of impairment.

American Medical Association

The 1984 American Medical Association[3] *Guides* in general follows the American Thoracic Society recommendations.[2] One departure is that the PaO_2 must be less than 50 Torr (versus 55 in the American Thoracic Society Statement) to be "itself a criterion for severe impairment." In addition, hypoxemia must be documented on two occasions, at least 4 weeks apart. An asthmatic patient is severely impaired when she has had episodes of bronchospasm requiring emergency room or hospital care on the average of 6 time a year despite optimum medical therapy.

The *Guides* provide criteria for partial impairments (Table 14-3). Mild impairment (Class 2), 10–25 percent, is present if dyspnea occurs when walking fast on the level ground or walking up a hill or stairs (grade 2 in Table 14-2) *or* the FVC or FEV_1 is below the lower 95 percent confidence interval (CI) but greater than 60 percent of predicted, *or* the FEV_1/FVC is below the CI but greater than 0.60 *or* the $\dot{V}O_{2max}$ is between 20–25 ml/kg/min. Moderate impairment (Class 3), 30–45 percent, is present if dyspnea occurs while walking on level ground with persons of the same age (grade 3) or up one flight of stairs, *or* FVC *or* FEV_1 is 50–59 percent of predicted *or* FEV_1/FVC is 0.40–0.59, *or* $\dot{V}O_{2max}$ is 15–20 ml/kg/min. Severe impairment (Class 4) is 50–100 percent and is present when dyspnea occurs after

Table 14-3
Classification of Respiratory Impairment

	Class 1 0% No Impairment	Class 2 10–25% Mild Impairment	Class 3 30–45% Moderate Impairment	Class 4 50–100% Severe Impairment
DYSPNEA	If dyspnea is present, it is consistent with the activity.	Dyspnea with fast walking on level ground or when walking up a hill; patient can keep pace with persons of same age and body build on level ground but not on hills or stairs.	Dyspnea while walking on level ground with person of the same age or walking up one flight of stairs. Patient can walk a mile at own pace.	Dyspnea after walking more than 100 meters at own pace on level ground. Patient sometimes is dyspneic with less exertion or even at rest.
	or	or	or	or
TESTS OF VENTILATORY FUNCTION				
FVC FEV_1 FEV_1/FVC ratio (as percent)	Above the lower limit of normal for the predicted value as defined by the 95% confidence interval.	Below the 95% confidence interval but greater than 60% predicted for FVC, FEV_1, and FEV_1/FVC ratio.	Less than 60% predicted, but greater than: 50% predicted for FVC 40% predicted for FEV_1 40% actual value for FEV_1/FVC ratio.	Less than: 50% predicted for FVC 40% predicted for FEV_1 40% actual value for FEV_1/FVC ratio 40% predicted for D_{co}.
	or	or	or	or
$\dot{V}O_2max$	Greater than 25 ml/(kg · min)	Between 20–25 ml/(kg · min)	Between 15–20 ml/(kg · min)	Less than 15 ml/(kg · min)

From American Medical Association. Guides to the Evaluation of Permanent Impairment (ed 2). Chicago, AMA, 1984, p 86, with permission.

236

walking 100 m at one's own pace on level ground (Grade 4), *or* FVC is less than 50 percent of predicted or FEV_1 is less than 40 percent of predicted, *or* FEV_1/FVC is less than 0.40, *or* standardized D_LCO_{SB} is less than 40 percent of predicted *or* VO_{2max} is less than 15 ml/kg/min.

The American Medical Association ratings permit combining partial impairments of two or more organ systems to arrive at a percentage impairment of the "whole person." "The principle is that each impairment acts not on the whole part but on the portion that remains after the preceding impairment has acted."

INTEGRATION OF CLINICAL AND LABORATORY FINDINGS

A major problem is how to compensate the claimant who has dyspnea and limitation of effort, who shows evidence of a respiratory disorder, and whose lung function is impaired but not to the marked degree required by most schemes. Exercise testing is one approach and is discussed in Chapter 15. For many such patients, clinical judgment, by integrating the medical, radiographic, and pulmonary function findings with knowledge of the natural history of the disease and of its course in that patient, may permit a fair assessment. A rapidly progressive interstitial pneumonitis poorly responsive to corticosteroid therapy should entitle an applicant to compensation even if his present pulmonary functions are above the cut-off limits. Similar lung volumes that have been unchanged for many years in a patient with fibrothorax following childhood empyema do not indicate the same prognosis.

For this intermediate group, breathing reserve ratio or observed response to standardized nonmaximal exercise (stair climbing; walk at a rapid pace) may be useful and provide semiquantitative data. These procedures are simple, universally available, and noninvasive.

References

1. Gaensler EA, Wright GW. Evaluation of respiratory impairment. Arch Environ Health 12:146–189, 1966
2. American Thoracic Society. Evaluation of impairment/disability secondary to respiratory disease. Am Rev Respir Dis 125:945–951, 1982
3. American Medical Association. Guides to the Evaluation of Permanent Impairment (ed 2). Chicago, AMA, 1984, pp 85–101
4. Snider GL, Kory RC, Lyons HA. Grading of pulmonary function impairment by means of pulmonary function tests. Recommendations of the Committee on Pulmonary Physiology, American College of Chest Physicians. Dis Chest 52:270–271, 1967
5. Morgan WKC. Pulmonary disability and impairment. Can't work? Won't work? Basics RD 10:5, 1982
6. American Medical Association, Committee on Rating of Mental and Physical Impairment. Guides to evaluation of permanent impairment. The respiratory system. JAMA 194:177–190, 1965

7. Mohler JG. Quantification of dyspnea confirmed by voice pitch analysis. Bull Physiopath Resp 18:837–850, 1982
8. Bowie DM, LeBlanc P, Killian KJ, et al. Can the intensity of breathlessness be predicted from the inspiratory flow rate? Am Rev Respir Dis 129:A239, 1984
9. Campbell EJM, Freedman S, Smith DS. The ability of man to detect added elastic loads to breathing. Clin Sci 20:223–231, 1961
10. Capel LH, Smart J. Obstructive airway disease. Measurements of effort intolerance and forced expiratory volume in bronchitis, emphysema, and asthma. Lancet 1:960–962, 1959
11. McGavin CR, Artivinli M, Nase H, et al. Dyspnea, disability and distance walked: Comparison of estimates of exercise performance in respiratory disease. Br Med J 2:241–243, 1978
12. American Thoracic Society. Evaluation of impairment/disability secondary to respiratory disorders. Am Rev Respir Dis 133:1205–1209, 1986
13. Social Security Administration. Disability evaluation under Social Security. A handbook for physicians. HEW Pub No. (SSA) 79-10089, August 1979

15

Incremental Exercise Testing (The Cardiorespiratory Stress Test)

David J. Kanarek
Albert Miller

USE IN ASSESSMENT OF IMPAIRMENT

The rationale of exercise tests is to determine the ability of the subject to meet the demands of his job. Tables are available that give the energy requirements of many tasks that can be matched against the actual measurements of the subject's exercise tolerance (Table 15-1).[1]

PULMONARY FUNCTION TESTS: A   ISBN 0-8089-1764-4   Copyright © 1987 by Grune & Stratton
GUIDE FOR THE STUDENT AND HOUSE OFFICER   All rights of reproduction in any form reserved.

Table 15-1
Energy Requirements of Various Activities

	$\dot{V}O_2$ (L/min)*
Personal Care	
Dressing and undressing	0.5–0.8
Shower, bath	0.5–0.8
Walking—2 mph	0.4–0.8
Climbing stairs	0.7–1.4
Recreation	
Tennis	1.5–2.0
Gardening	1.0–2.0
Cycling—5 mph	0.8–1.0
Cycling—13 mph	2.0
Bowling	0.9–1.2
Skiing	2.0–4.0
Domestic Work	
Sweeping	0.4
Scrubbing	0.8–1.2
Making beds	0.8–1.0
Washing clothes	0.8–1.0
Occupation	
Desk	0.3–0.4
Bricklaying	0.8
Benchwork	0.4–0.5
Coal mining	0.8–2.0
Agriculture	0.6–1.8
Heavy manual work	1.5–2.5
Snow shoveling	3.5
Lumberjack	1.5–4.0

*for a 70 kg man.

It is important to appreciate that exercise testing is carried out in a laboratory for a brief period of time, 8 to 15 minutes. It does not directly measure endurance, or the effect of environmental factors such as high temperature or humidity, which may affect performance under working conditions.

Other factors such as age, obesity, duration of exercise, and specificity of training for the work all affect the ability to perform a job. An obese individual with the same $\dot{V}O_{2max}$ as a lean subject may need to expend more of her capacity moving her own body, leaving less capacity for the task at hand.

Exercise studies define the functional capacity of an individual. Broad categories that impair exercise tolerance include pulmonary disease, cardiac disease, poor physical fitness, and peripheral muscle weakness (Table 15-2). Several of these factors may be present simultaneously. In particular, deconditioning, in which lack of exercise leads to loss of functional capacity (Fig. 15-1), frequently accompanies

Table 15-2
Patterns of Response in Exercise tests

	Cardiac Disease	Obstructive Lung Disease	Interstitial Lung Disease	Deconditioned
$\dot{V}O_2$ (max)	↓	↓↓	↓↓	↓
$\dot{V}_E$/MVV	N	↑	↑	N
HR (max) % pred	80%	80%	80%	N/↑
O_2 pulse (max)	↓	↓↓	↓	N/↓
VD/VT	N	↑	↑	N
AT	↓	↓	↓	N
PaO_2 (rest)	N	↓	↓↓	N
(peak exercise)	N/↑	↓/↓↓	↓↓	N

Legend: N = within normal range; ↓ = small decrease; ↓↓ = marked decrease; ↑ = increase

organic disease of any etiology. Definition of the pathology producing the impairment, with the notable exception of ischemic heart disease, usually depends upon studies at rest: the *effect* of the disease is measured during exercise.

Patterns of Response

These responses have been obtained by studying subjects with as "pure" a disease state as possible. It should be realized, however, that combinations are frequent. For example, emphysema or ILD also involves the pulmonary vasculature, which in turn, may impair right ventricular function.

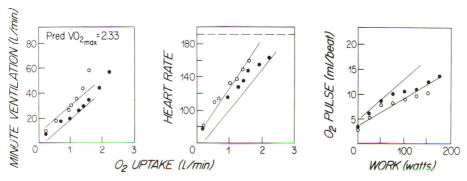

Fig. 15-1. The effect of a 3-month jogging program on a healthy 30-year-old woman; before (open circles), after (closed circles). Note lower $\dot{V}_E$ and HR and higher O_2 pulse after training. O_2 pulse = $\dot{V}O_2$/HR.

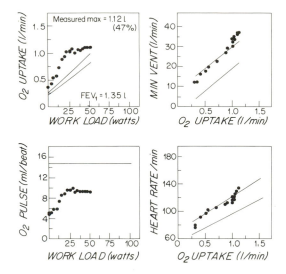

Fig. 15-2. A 58-year-old man with severe aortic regurgitation demonstrates the pattern of cardiovascular dysfunction. $\dot{V}O_2$ max is reduced with a plateau, AT is <1 L/min $\dot{V}O_2$, O_2 pulse is reduced and HR is at upper limits of normal. In all figures solid lines indicate range of predicted values.

Pattern of Cardiac Dysfunction

(See Fig. 15-2)

Decreased $\dot{V}O_{2max}$, with frequent plateau formation

Reduced anaerobic threshold (AT) as a percentage of predicted $\dot{V}O_{2max}$; AT remains in proportion to decrease in $\dot{V}O_{2max}$

Reduced O_2 pulse

High heart rate

V_D/V_T falls normally

PaO_2 shows no change or increases with exercise

Pattern of Ventilatory Dysfunction

(See Fig. 15-3)

Elevated $\dot{V}O_{Emax}/MVV$

High respiratory rate

Decreased peak $\dot{V}O_2$, without plateau formation

In obstructive disease AT is absent or occurs close to peak $\dot{V}O_2$

V_D/V_T may be elevated at rest and does not fall normally (in emphysema and ILD)

PaO_2 falls (in emphysema and ILD)

Pattern of Pulmonary Vascular Disease

(See Fig. 15-4)

Increased V_D/V_T ratio at rest that does not fall with exercise

Decreased $\dot{V}O_{2max}$

Reduced AT

High heart rate

Increased $\dot{V}O_E$

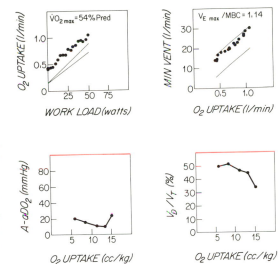

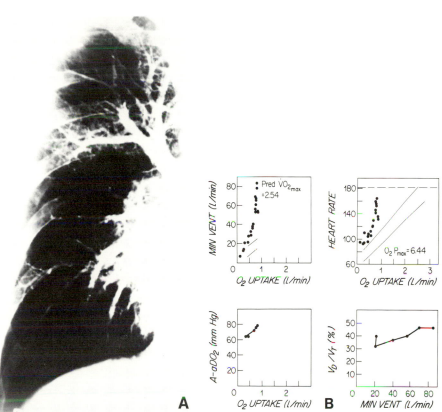

Fig. 15-3. A 60-year-old male with severe CAO (FEV_1 1.1 L) demonstrates the pattern of ventilatory dysfunction: $\dot{V}O_2$ max is reduced. $\dot{V}_E$ max is greater than 100 percent of MVV, no AT is seen though lactate level was 4.2 mEq at peak exercise, and V_D/V_T is elevated and does not fall normally.

Fig. 15-4. (A) Pulmonary angiogram showing severe vascular obstruction due to pulmonary emboli. (B) Same patient as in (A) demonstrating the pattern of pulmonary vascular disease: very high $\dot{V}_E$ and very early AT, elevated HR, elevated $P(A-a)O_2$ at rest increasing further with exercise and high V_D/V_T at rest, increasing further with exercise.

243

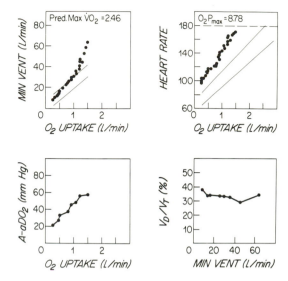

Fig. 15-5. A 46-year-old male with severe interstitial fibrosis who demonstrates a reduced $\dot{V}O_2$ max, a relatively early AT at $\dot{V}O_2$ 1.2 L/min, a high HR, a reduced O_2 pulse, a progressive increase in $P(A-a)O_2$ and an elevated V_D/V_T at rest and exercise.

Figure 15-5 shows the exercise responses of a patient with severe ILD. These patients typically incorporate features of all three patterns of dysfunction since there may be a reduction in ventilatory capacity, the pulmonary vasculature is inevitably involved and pulmonary artery pressure is elevated, affecting the right ventricle.

ENERGY REQUIREMENTS OF VARIOUS ACTIVITIES

There is a body of knowledge concerning the energy demands of certain jobs and sporting activities (Table 15-1). Given that resting oxygen consumption is approximately 250 ml/min (1 MET) or 3.5 ml/kg/min, a broad classification of work load is useful:

Light work $<.5$ L/min (2 MET)

Moderate $.5 - 1.0$ L/min (2–4 MET)

Moderately heavy $1.0 - 1.9$ L/min (6–8 MET)

Extremely heavy ≥ 2.0 L/min (≥ 8 METS)

The ability to achieve increasing levels of oxygen uptake depends on the integrity of the cardiopulmonary system to supply sufficient oxygenated blood to the exercising muscles. An individual may be limited by reduction in ventilatory capacity, oxygen transfer or cardiac output, inappropriate distribution of cardiac output, or limited peripheral extraction of oxygen. Exercise testing is capable of measuring these variables.

Jones[2] provides equations for predicting maximal power output:

Equation 15-1a

$$\text{Males (kpm/min)}^* = 25.3 \text{ Ht(cm)} - 9.06 \text{ Age (yrs)} - 2759$$

Equation 15-1b

$$\text{Females (kpm/min)}^* = 9.5 \text{ Ht(cm)} - 9.21 \text{ Age (yrs)} + 6.1 \text{ Wt (kg)} - 756$$

$$^*\text{Watts} = \frac{\text{Kpm/min}}{6}$$

MAXIMUM OXYGEN UPTAKE ($\dot{V}O_{2max}$)

This is the "gold standard" that requires maximum effort from the subject. Generally, an individual can utilize no more than about 30–40 percent of the maximum oxygen uptake continually during an 8-hour working day, without experiencing fatigue.[3] However, short bursts requiring the use of up to 100 percent of full aerobic capacity can be tolerated.[4] The percentage of maximum capacity that can be sustained ranges from 64 percent for work duration of 1 hour to 33 percent for 8 hours.[5,6]

There is a linear relationship between $\dot{V}O_2$ and work load. The true maximum $\dot{V}O_2$ ($\dot{V}O_{2max}$) is that point at which an increasing work load no longer elicits an increase in $\dot{V}O_2$, ie, a plateau is reached. This feature is usually not seen in normal subjects when a bicycle is used.

A plateau is characteristically present when a patient with moderately severe cardiac disease exercises on a bicycle. It is not present with predominant lung disease. When a plateau is not present, "peak $\dot{V}O_2$" or "symptomatic $\dot{V}O_{2max}$" should be used to describe the highest VO_2 achieved.

Equation 15-2a (Jones[7])

$$\text{Predicted } \dot{V}O_{2max} \text{ (L/min)} = 4.2 - 0.032 \text{ age (males)}$$

Equation 15-2b (Jones[7])

$$\text{Predicted } \dot{V}O_{2max} \text{ (L/min)} = 2.8 - 0.014 \text{ age (females)}$$

Predicted values provide a comparison between the subject's performance and those of equivalent sex, height, and age. However, unlike resting pulmonary function tests in which comparison between actual and predicted values is useful for determining presence and degree of impairment, in exercise studies the actual value of oxygen uptake is important. This is because the appropriate comparison is not to a "normal" person, but to the oxygen uptake required to carry out a specific task.

VENTILATORY ANAEROBIC THRESHOLD (AT)

When progressive exercise is performed, minute ventilation increases linearly and then increases out of proportion to the increase in oxygen uptake.[8,9] This point indicates the ventilatory AT and correlates with a concurrent increase in lactate levels in the blood and the development of metabolic acidosis. There is a relation between the development of fatigue during exercise and acidosis, though this does not necessarily imply a direct link. The ventilatory AT is best visualized graphically by plotting the minute ventilation or derivatives thereof such as the ventilatory equivalent for O_2 ($\dot{V}_E/\dot{V}O_2$) against work load or $\dot{V}O_2$ in an incremental study.[8,9] The AT occurs at 50–65 percent of the observed maximum oxygen uptake in untrained subjects. It may be delayed to > 80 percent of the observed $\dot{V}O_{2max}$ in either highly trained individuals (because they are efficient) or those with very poor exercise performance (because they can barely surpass the anaerobic threshold). Very large differences in both $\dot{V}O_{2max}$ and the level at which AT occurs separate these two groups. The AT may also be related to the predicted $\dot{V}O_{2max}$; a ratio >40 percent is considered normal.

The AT is an important marker identifying a level of work that cannot be exceeded if performance is to be maintained. Short bursts of work can exceed this level, provided there is a subsequent reduction in activity that allows recovery to take place.

MINUTE VENTILATION ($\dot{V}_E$)

Progressive exercise is accompanied by a linear increase in $\dot{V}_E$, up to the AT. A reduction in the maximum capacity for ventilation, either by obstructive or restrictive disease, may limit exercise. The upper limit to ventilation is reasonably estimated by $FEV_1 \times 35$–40.

Any subject who requires more than 50 percent of his maximal capacity for ventilation to carry out a task will have grounds for claiming dyspnea. The ratio of $\dot{V}_{Emax}/MBC$ (predicted from the FEV_1) was 0.69 in normal subjects studied by Mahler et al.[10] and very high in patients with CAO (may exceed 1.0).

The $\dot{V}_E$ at a given $\dot{V}O_2$ (or work load) may be a simple, noninvasive criterion to evaluate the respiratory response to exercise.[11]

The ventilatory equivalent for oxygen (the amount of ventilation required to extract a given amount of O_2, $\dot{V}_E/\dot{V}O_2$), is sometimes suggested as an estimate of the efficiency of ventilation. Subjects with lung disease have a higher $\dot{V}_E$ and $\dot{V}_E/\dot{V}O_2$ than normal subjects relative to work load, because of increased dead space ventilation, hypoxemia and other poorly characterized factors such as pulmonary hypertension.

HEART RATE (HR)

There is a linear relationship between $\dot{V}O_2$ and HR. Stroke volume reaches a maximum in normal individuals at a HR of approximately 120/min; cardiac output increases thereafter by an increase in HR. The maximum HR can be estimated by the following formulae (See also Figure 12-7):

Equation 15-3a[7]

$$HR\ max = 220 - age\ (years)$$

Equation 15-3b[7]

$$HR\ max = 210 - 0.65 \times age\ (years)$$

With increasing age there is, therefore, a decrease in maximum cardiac output and a decrease in $\dot{V}O_{2max}$.

The slope of the relationship $HR:\dot{V}O_2$ is steeper in myocardial disease where the reduced SV is compensated for by an increase HR to maintain Q and thereby meet the O_2 demands of the exercising muscles; Q and therefore exercise performance are limited by the HR reaching a maximum early in the exercise stint.

Achievement of 85 percent of the predicted maximum HR indicates an adequate effort and correlates with a level 75 percent to 85 percent of the $\dot{V}O_{2max}$ in a normal subject.

O_2 PULSE

The O_2 pulse, $\dot{V}O_2/HR$, can be derived from the Fick principle for measurement of cardiac output:

Equation 15-4

$$\dot{V}O_2/HR = SV \times (a-\bar{v})DO_2$$

where SV = stroke volume; HR = heart rate and $(a-\bar{v})DO_2$ is the difference in O_2 content between arterial and mixed venous blood.

A reduced O_2 pulse may reflect either a relatively low stroke volume with a compensatory elevation in heart rate to maintain an appropriate cardiac output for the level of exercise, or limited peripheral extraction of O_2 reducing the $\dot{V}O_2$, which is seen in sepsis. In congestive heart failure, on the other hand, peripheral extraction is increased, widening the arterial-mixed venous DO_2 and counteracting the decrease in SV. Despite this compensatory increase in $a-\bar{v}\ DO_2$, the O_2 pulse is generally low. The O_2 pulse cannot differentiate between these central and peripheral mechanisms. Consideration of the clinical circumstances is helpful, however; in the majority of cases the stroke volume will be at fault.

ARTERIAL BLOOD GASES

A marked fall in PaO_2 during exercise is typical of ILD and emphysema. The PaO_2 may rise on exercise when ventilation-perfusion relationships improve in chronic bronchitis, asthma, and obesity. An increase in $PaCO_2$ on exercise may be seen in patients with CAO.[12]

DEAD SPACE VENTILATION (V_D/V_T)

The normal resting value for V_D/V_T is 30–42 percent depending on age. With exercise, the V_D/V_T falls rapidly, reaching between 20 and 25 percent by the time about 1 liter $\dot{V}O_2$ or 50 watts has been reached. Thereafter it continues to fall more slowly and may reach levels as low as 10 percent.[13] It is, however, the initial fall or lack thereof that is most helpful. The normal fall in V_D/V_T reflects an increased efficiency of ventilation and is due to the increase in tidal volume being distributed largely to well perfused areas of the lungs. When lung regions are ventilated but not perfused, as for example, in pulmonary embolic disease, part of the increase in tidal volume may be distributed to the nonperfused areas, reducing or eliminating the fall in V_D/V_T.

The V_D/V_T has been found to be a useful indicator of pulmonary vascular disease. An elevated V_D/V_T frequently provides the explanation for an elevated $\dot{V}_E$ during exercise in lung disease. Its presence in emphysema and ILD reflects damage to the capillaries which is an inevitable concomitant of these diseases. It should be noted that the V_D/V_T, reflecting areas of high $\dot{V}/\dot{Q}$, does not necessarily parallel other gas exchange abnormalities. For example, there may be no fall in PaO_2 with exercise despite a high V_D/V_T and vice versa, an abnormal fall in PaO_2 may be associated with a normal fall in V_D/V_T.

SIMPLE TESTS OF EXERCISE CAPABILITY

Such assessments as walking two flights of stairs, self-paced walking over a fixed course[14] or the maximum distance that can be walked in 12 minutes[15] may supplement clinical evaluation (see Chapter 14, *Integration of clinical and laboratory findings*).

One of the oldest exercise assessments used by pulmonologists is the step stool test, with the goal of completing 30 step-ups (equivalent to two flights of stairs) in 60 to 120 seconds. This has been found useful to detect a fall in PaO_2 in ILD, even if the latter is not radiographically evident; falls are not seen in normal subjects or those with chest wall restriction.[16] There is a rough correlation among symptoms, step-up ability, and response to progressive exercise in CAO. A patient able to walk briskly on the level can usually complete 30 step-ups without difficulty and achieve a $\dot{V}O_{2max} > 1.5$ L/min. One who must walk slowly on level ground can complete the

30 step-ups only by becoming dyspneic and has a VO_{2max} between 1.0 and 1.5 L/min. A patient who must stop on level ground cannot complete 30 step-ups or reach a $\dot{V}O_{2max}$ of 1.0 L/min.

PROTOCOLS FOR EXERCISE TESTING

Either a treadmill or a cycle ergometer is suitable for producing graded loads. Treadmill walking is more familiar and also produces the highest measured $\dot{V}O_{2max}$. The cycle, while less familiar, has less training effect, causes fewer mishaps and permits arterial blood samples to be obtained more easily.

The American Lung Association Committee in Disability[17] has recommended that the initial study be carried out by Jones' technique in which the subject begins exercising on a cycle at 100 kilopondmeters (KPM)/min (ca. 16 watts), increasing the load by 50 to 100 KPM/min, while measurements of ventilation and HR are made. The $\dot{V}O_2$ is not measured directly but can be calculated from simple equations, knowing the power output:[17]

Equation 15-5

$$\dot{V}O_2 \text{ ml/min} = 2 \times \text{power output (KPM/min)} + \text{basal } O_2 \text{ uptake}$$

where basal O_2 uptake $= 3.5 \times$ wt in kg. In addition, plots of ventilation against power output may permit the AT to be recognized. If this test is equivocal, further measurements such as actual $\dot{V}O_2$, arterial blood gases and dead space to tidal volume ratios are recommended.

This protocol has the advantage of a simple initial test. However, the measurement of oxygen uptake directly is not very complex with commercial equipment now available. Carbon dioxide can be measured at the same time, allowing the ventilatory equivalents for oxygen and carbon dioxide and the "R" value to be recorded. These measurements enable the AT to be recognized more easily. Arterial blood gases and therefore, V_D/V_T and $P(A-a)O_2$, are of use in explaining unexpected hyperventilation or a major inconsistency between resting and exercise values, as may occur in pulmonary vascular disease or ILD.

ILLUSTRATIVE CASES

Case 15-1

A 47-year-old, 6-foot-tall automobile mechanic complained of grade II dyspnea. He had smoked 30 pack years and had a mild congestive cardiomyopathy. Physical examination showed prolonged expiration, decreased breath sounds, and no evidence of congestive heart failure. Chest x-ray showed hyperinflated lungs and slight cardiomegaly. Pulmonary function studies follow:

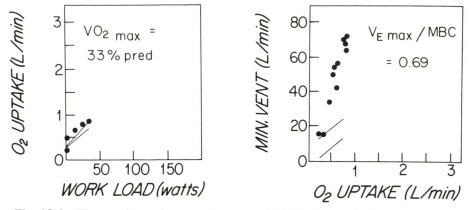

Fig. 15-6. The exercise performance in a man with ILD. Set text for interpretation. The straight lines delineate the predicted response.

FEV$_1$ 1.21 (26% pred)
FVC 3.80L (77% pred)
FEV$_1$/FVC 0.31

(No BD response, and no improvement after therapy).

Comment

This man had severe CAO, fulfilling various criteria for complete disability. Exercise studies were not needed.

Case 15-2

A 57-year-old truck driver complained of grade III dyspnea when loading his truck; he had smoked 30 pack years. Physical examination showed bilateral basal crackles, and chest x-ray showed a diffuse process, which lung biopsy demonstrated to be interstitial fibrosis. Pulmonary function studies follow:

FEV$_1$ 2.99 L (90% pred)
FVC 3.78L (88% pred)
D$_L$CO$_{SB}$ 16.2 ml/min/mm Hg (64% pred)

These data were out of proportion to the degree of dyspnea and an exercise study was carried out (Fig. 15-6). The $\dot{V}O_{2max}$ was 0.8 liters (33 percent of predicted), the AT occurred at a $\dot{V}O_2$ of 0.5 liters and the PO$_2$ decreased to 50 mm Hg. The $\dot{V}_E$ increased dramatically and reached 69 percent of MBC. An electrocardiogram during the study demonstrated depression of ST segments.

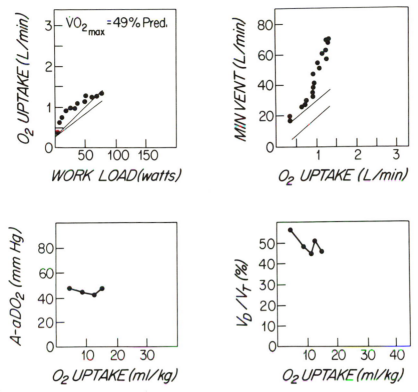

Fig. 15-7. Measurements during exercise in a fireman with mild CAO and reduced DL. See text for interpretation; note that P(A-a)O$_2$, shown as A-a DO$_2$ in the figure, is high throughout and that V$_D$/V$_T$ is markedly elevated at rest and does not fall normally. The straight lines delineate the predicted response.

Comment

The exercise study demonstrated severe impairment of exercise tolerance, showing the typical features of ILD. The early AT may have been contributed to by the myocardial ischemia. Resting pulmonary function values grossly underestimated the exercise limitation.

Case 15-3

A 54-year-old fireman claimed that he was unable to carry out his duties without severe dyspnea. He had smoked 30 pack years and had a daily nonproductive cough. Physical examination showed moderate wheezing. Pulmonary function studies at rest were:

FEV_1 2.41 (74% of pred)
FVC 3.50 L (85% pred)
D_LCO_{SB} 15.4 ml/min/mm Hg (52% pred)

An exercise study was performed (Fig. 15-7).

Comment

The exercise study showed a marked reduction in $\dot{V}O_{2max}$ to 1.4 liters as well as an AT occurring at 1 liter $\dot{V}O_2$. Note the long period of anaerobic exercise demonstrating the effort made. The ratio $\dot{V}_E/MVV$ reached 75 percent at maximum exercise, a level associated with dyspnea. At AT, however, $\dot{V}_E$ was only 32 L/min. or a $\dot{V}_E/MVV$ of 33 percent, a level below that associated with dyspnea. In this patient, the capacity to work is reduced, but at AT this is not due to ventilatory limitation. The lower two panels of Figure 15-7 demonstrate elevated V_D/V_T and $P(A-a)O_2$. These features explain the higher ventilatory requirement and provide at least a partial explanation for the reduction in working capacity.

References

1. Wiedemann HP, Gee JBL, Balmes JR, et al. Exercise testing in occupational lung diseases. Clin Chest Med 5:157–171, 1984
2. Jones NL, Makrides L, Hitchcock C, et al. Normal standards for an incremental progressive cycle ergometer test. Am Rev Respir Dis 131:700–708, 1985
3. Astrand PO. Quantification of exercise capability and evaluation of physical capacity in man. Prog Cardiovasc Dis 19:51–67, 1976
4. Astrand PO, Rodahl K. Textbook of Work Physiology. New York: McGraw-Hill, 1977, pp 299–301
5. Erb BD. Applying work physiology to occupational medicine. Occup Health Safety 50:20–24, 1981
6. Bonjer FH. Actual energy expenditure in relation to physical working capacity. Ergonomics 5:29–31, 1962
7. Jones NL, Campbell EJ, Edwards RHT, et al. Clinical Exercise Testing (ed 2). Philadelphia, WB Saunders, 1982
8. Wasserman K, Whipp BJ, Koyal SN, et al. Anaerobic threshold and respiratory gas exchange during exercise. J Appl Physiol 34:236–243, 1973
9. Wasserman K. The anaerobic threshold measurement to evaluate exercise performance. Am Rev Respir Dis 129 (suppl):35–40, 1984
10. Mahler DA, Moritz ED, Loke J. Exercise performance in marathon runners. Med Sci Sport Ex 13:284–289, 1981
11. Spiro SG. Exercise testing in clinical medicine. Br J Dis Chest 71:145–172, 1977
12. Nery LE, Wasserman K, French W, et al. Contrasting cardiovascular and respiratory responses to exercise in mitral valve and chronic obstructive pulmonary diseases. Chest 83:446–453, 1983
13. Jones NL, McHardy GJR, Naimark A, et al. Physiological deadspace and alveolar-arterial gas pressures during exercise. Clin Sci 31:19–29, 1966

14. Bassey EJ, Fentem PH, MacDonald IC, et al. Self paced walking as a method for exercise testing in elderly and young men. Clin Sci Mol Med 51:609–612, 1976

15. McGavin CR, Artivinli M, Nase H, et al. Dyspnea, disability and distance walked: Comparison of estimates of exercise performance in respiratory disease. Br Med J 2:241–243, 1978

16. Morrison D, Kory R, Goldman A. The step test in interstitial lung disease. Chest 74:345, 1978

17. American Thoracic Society. Evaluation of impairment/disability secondary to respiratory disease. Am Rev Respir Dis 5:945–951, 1982

16

Sleep and Breathing

David M. Rapoport

Respiration During Normal Sleep
  Non-REM Sleep
  REM Sleep
  Effect of Sleep on Upper Airway and Chest Cage Muscles
Patterns of Abnormal Respiration During Sleep
  Obstructive Sleep Apnea (OSA)
  Central Sleep Apnea (CSA)
  Cheyne-Stokes Respiration
Monitoring of Respiration
  Ventilation
    Qualitative Detection of Respiratory Air Flow
    Quantitation
  Respiratory Effort
  Consequences of Respiratory Events
Case Histories
  Obstructive Sleep Apnea
  Central Sleep Apnea

PULMONARY FUNCTION TESTS: A   ISBN 0-8089-1764-4   Copyright © 1987 by Grune & Stratton
GUIDE FOR THE STUDENT AND HOUSE OFFICER   All rights of reproduction in any form reserved.

RESPIRATION DURING NORMAL SLEEP

Any discussion of sleep must begin with an understanding of the state itself, which is not uniform.[1] Sleep consists of a highly organized sequence of sub-states, which can be broadly separated into Rapid Eye Movement (REM) and non-Rapid Eye Movement (non-REM) sleep.[2] These are defined by a constellation of electro-encephalographic (EEG) and behavioral criteria. Non-REM sleep is further divided into light (stages I and II) and deep (stages III and IV) sleep.

Non-REM Sleep

This state is perhaps closest to the lay conception of "restful sleep." It has been likened to "a sleeping brain in a responsive body." During this state, metabolic activity is reduced, ventilation and heart rate tend to be slow and regular, skeletal muscle tone is mildly diminished and cerebral activity is reduced. Physiologic control mechanisms are similar to those present during the waking state. Overall ventilation drops slightly and arterial PCO_2 rises 2–3 Torr.[3-5]

REM Sleep

Rather than an extreme in a continuum of "sleep," REM sleep is a very different physiologic state.[2,3] It has been likened to "an awake brain in an unresponsive body." Cerebral activity is intense and brain metabolic demands may actually rise.[6] On the other hand, a nearly total suppression of skeletal muscular tone occurs sparing only the eye muscles and the diaphragm.[2] This suppression affects many of the respiratory muscles, including the muscles of the upper airway (see below). Episodes of REM sleep last 20–30 minutes, occur every 90 to 120 minutes during normal sleep[2] and are longest in the early morning. They alternate with periods of approximately 1 hour of non-REM sleep. During REM sleep physiologic functions including heart rate, blood pressure and respiration are irregular[7] and may respond only partially to the usual external stimuli.[2] It is during REM sleep that dreams occur.[8] Ventilatory responses to inspired CO_2 are markedly reduced[9]; there may also be a reduction in response to hypoxia.[10] In addition, arousal from sleep itself is markedly blunted: levels of hypoxia,[10,11] hypercapnia,[9] or laryngeal stimulation[12,13] that resulted in arousal from non-REM sleep are not sufficient to produce arousal from REM sleep.

Effect of Sleep on Upper Airway and Chest Cage Muscles

During wakefulness, normal breathing consists of a highly coordinated sequence of contractions of the muscles of respiration.[14,15] A baseline level of muscle tone maintains patency in the upper airway; this tone disappears only during swallowing. Just before contraction of the diaphragm at the onset of each breath, a neural discharge causes contraction of the muscles of the upper airway.[16] This causes the pharyngeal walls to further stiffen while contraction of the genioglossal muscle pushes the tongue forward. Patency of the upper airway is maintained by thus stabilizing it against collapse due to the negative intraluminal pressures of inspiration.[15] The intercostal muscles are then activated to stabilize the chest wall.[17] Finally the diaphragm contracts and generates the negative intrathoracic pressure which moves air during inspiration.[18]

Loss of any part of this orderly sequence of muscle activity can impair ventilation. Failure of the upper airway muscles to contract and become rigid will result in a tendency to passive collapse during inspiration.[19] Failure of the intercostal muscles to contract to stabilize the chest wall will result in paradoxical (inward) movement during inspiration, dissipating the negative pressure generated by the diaphragm.[20] Finally, failure of the diaphragm to contract adequately and descend will impair the generation of negative intrathoracic pressure. During REM sleep there is a profound inhibition of baseline tone of most skeletal muscles which also affects the muscles of the upper airway and the intercostals.[14,21] The loss of pharyngeal tone predisposes to airway collapse on inspiration. Loss of baseline genioglossal tone causes displacement of the tongue posteriorly narrowing the airway. Loss of intercostal muscle tone leads to instability of the chest wall during inspiration; paradoxical (inward) inspiratory chest movements occur frequently during REM sleep. In addition to decreased baseline tone, the phasic inspiratory discharges of the upper airway and intercostal muscles may be inhibited during REM sleep,[14,19] leaving the upper airway and chest wall further destabilized while the diaphragm is left unaided in generating inspiratory pressures. Ineffective or obstructed ventilation is thus most likely in REM sleep during the very time when arousal and responses to other stimuli are most depressed.

PATTERNS OF ABNORMAL RESPIRATION
DURING SLEEP

Obstructive Sleep Apnea (OSA)

In the adult population the syndrome characterized by obstructive apneas is the most prevalent respiratory disorder recognized during sleep.[22] The diagnosis is established by demonstrating the presence of apneas (or absence of air movement) lasting more than 10 seconds, accompanied by persisting respiratory effort.[23] In order to be clearly abnormal, there must be more than 5 apneas per hour of sleep or more than 15 in a night, some of which must be in non-REM sleep. The disorder is primarily seen in obese subjects without other disease.[23] However it also occurs in the nonobese,[23] and may be associated with hypothyroidism,[24] acromegaly,[25] and congenital or acquired abnormalities causing narrowing of the upper airway, such as tonsilar and adenoidal hypertrophy[26] or micrognathia.[27,28] Occasionally tumors of the upper airway,[29] or diffuse edema such as that due to superior vena caval obstruction, may produce obstructive sleep apnea. There may be little or no apparent airway impairment while the patient is awake.[23] In children the most common cause of the syndrome is tonsilar and adenoidal hypertrophy.[30]

The obstructions of the airway (apneas) result in periods of hypoventilation and arterial oxygen desaturation which occur repeatedly as soon as the patient sleeps (stage II sleep). These in turn cause momentary arousals which terminate each apnea. As a result of these periodic arousals the patient is sleep deprived and hypersomnolent during the day.[31] The patient is generally unaware of waking up, but may complain of insomnia. During an arousal, breathing may be normal or it may be partially obstructed. These partial obstructions account for the loud snoring and grunting characteristic of "sleep" in OSA.[32]

During the apneas respiratory efforts continue despite the patient's inability to move air past the collapsed upper airway. Intrathoracic pressure undergoes extreme fluctuations, reaching negative pressures approaching 80 cm H_2O. Vagal reflexes induced by these pressure changes (amounting to a Müller maneuver) and by variations in venous return contribute to the frequent arrhythmias seen during sleep in patients with OSA.[33,34]

In its most severe form, OSA is associated with incapacitating daytime hypersomnolence: this is frequently the patient's chief complaint.[31] Chronic hypercapnia (persisting while the patient is awake) may occur but is not the rule.[35] Right-sided heart failure is also seen.[36] Obstructive sleep apnea should be suspected in any patient (especially if obese) who presents with hypersomnolence or unexplained cardiorespiratory failure.

Central Sleep Apnea (CSA)

This syndrome is much less frequent but may overlap in the individual patient with OSA.[25] Central apneas are defined by a 10 second pause in air movement *not* associated with respiratory efforts.[23] They may occur during any stage of sleep but are clearly abnormal only in non-REM sleep.[25] The syndrome of central apnea may occur as an isolated abnormality or it may occur in association with a variety of disorders of the central nervous system including surgical trauma,[37] tumor,[38] infarction, or infection[39,40] affecting the brainstem. Central sleep apneas clearly represent an abnormality in central respiratory control mechanisms,[1] but a waking abnormality is not necessarily present.[41] Some patients with central sleep apnea do have the alveolar hypoventilation syndrome, "Ondine's Curse" (ie, chronic hypercapnia without intrinsic lung disease).[42] (See Chapter 10, Respiratory Center Unresponsiveness).

Cheyne-Stokes Respiration

This form of respiratory periodicity with pauses is seen in patients with low cardiac output, various diseases of the central nervous system, and in some normal elderly subjects.[1] The breath size modulates smoothly from small to large, then back to small before an apnea. By contrast, in central apnea onset of breathing tends to be abrupt and is often associated with an arousal. In addition, apneic periods in

Cheyne-Stokes breathing tend to be shorter, whereas central apneas may last in excess of 60 seconds.

MONITORING OF RESPIRATION

Ventilation

Qualitative Detection of Respiratory Air Flow

Demonstrating effective ventilation depends on sensing respiratory airflow at the mouth and/or nose. A simple device consists of a loosely fitted surgical *face mask* covering nose and mouth into which a tube with multiple openings is glued.[43] The tube is led to a pressure transducer, and the *pressure swings* recorded.

A small *sampling cannula* within or near the nares and/or mouth measures CO_2 or O_2 concentration in the exhaled gas. Alternatively, a *thermistor* can be clipped to the nose or lip, and will sense *temperature change.*

Quantitation

Of all the methods of quantitating ventilation, the one most generally useful and acceptable to the patient is the inductance plethysmograph, (Fig. 16-1) described below.

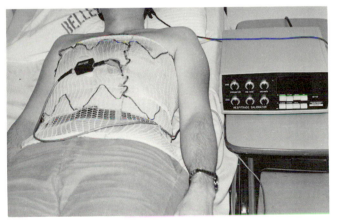

Fig. 16-1. Inductance plethysmograph (Respitrace, Ambulatory Monitoring, Ardsley, NY). Note coils around abdomen and chest which pick up changes in cross sectional area. These can be electronically scaled and added to give a signal proportional to actual tidal volume.

Respiratory Effort

Assessment of respiratory effort is necessary to differentiate central from obstructive apneas. This may be done by *direct observation* of movements of the patient's chest or abdomen during periods of absent airflow (apnea). Alternatively, *motion detectors* (eg, *strain gauges, magnetometers, or impedance probes*) can be placed on the chest and abdomen. The *inductance plethymograph* relies on the stretching of a mesh vest that changes the inductance of two electrical coils embedded in the vest and placed over the chest and abdomen, respectively. If the electrical signals are related to a particular patient's body habitus by a calibration procedure[44], ventilation can be measured with an accuracy within 10 percent. When chest, abdomen, and sum signals are recorded, this single device will provide detection of apnea and hypoventilation, and in most cases will differentiate obstructive from central apnea. Paradoxic movement of the chest and abdomen will be noted in the former and no respiratory movements in the latter.

Direct measurement of intrathoracic pressure is sometimes useful. A small catheter with a balloon at its tip is passed transnasally, positioned in the mid esophagus and connected to a pressure transducer. Negative pressure is a direct reflection of respiratory effort.

Consequences of Respiratory Events

The consequences of apnea and hypoventilation include transient but profound disturbances in arterial oxygenation and cardiac arrhythmias, as well as variable hypercapnia. The first two of these may be the most serious consequences of sleep-related abnormalities in breathing, and thus monitoring of ECG and arterial oxygenation are necessary. The latter is most easily done with an ear or finger oximeter.

CASE PRESENTATIONS

Obstructive Sleep Apnea

A 52-year-old obese male presents with a history of severe hypersomnolence. He falls asleep repeatedly during the interview. His wife reports "room-rocking" snoring with periods of silence interspersed, during which she has actually awakened him to "see if he was alive." Physical examination is remarkable only for obesity and the hypersomnolence noted above. The patient undergoes over-night sleep monitoring. A portion of the tracing is shown in Figure 16-2.

The patient has frequent cessations in airflow (both the mouth and nose channels show no deflection). During these periods the inductance plethysmograph shows persistent movement of the chest and abdomen, indicating that the apneas are obstructive. Note the paradoxical movements of the chest and abdomen channels during the apneas, in contrast to their parallel movement during unobstructed respiration. The consequences of each apnea are seen in the ear oximeter tracing. The lowest saturation occurs after breathing resumes. This is because of the circulation time needed for the desaturated blood from the lungs to arrive at the ear.

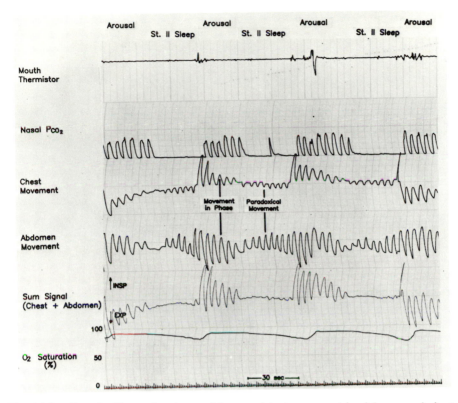

Fig. 16-2. Case 1. Obstructive Apnea. Note persistent movement in abdomen and chest sensors (Respitrace), with absent air flow at mouth (thermistor tracing flat) and nose (no CO_2 detected). The chest and abdomen movements are in opposite directions (paradoxical) during an apnea, whereas they are in phase during unobstructed breathing. Also note the desaturation which occurs with each apnea; lag is largely due to the circulation time from lung to ear.

Weight loss was recommended and resulted in a decrease in the number of apneas until the patient regained the weight one year later.

Central Sleep Apnea

A 45-year-old man presents with a history of muscular dystrophy, obesity, loud snoring, and hypersomnolence. On physical examination, the patient is obese and has profound muscular weakness of the arms, mild weakness of the legs, but good respiratory movements. His pulmonary function shows: vital capacity 70 percent of predicted, functional residual capacity 75 percent of predicted, maximum voluntary ventilation 62 percent of predicted and no evidence of airway obstruction. His PCO_2 is elevated (47 Torr) with a normal pH.

A full sleep study is done. A portion of the tracing (during stage II sleep) is shown in Figure 16-3. This shows apneas (no movement in either mouth thermistor

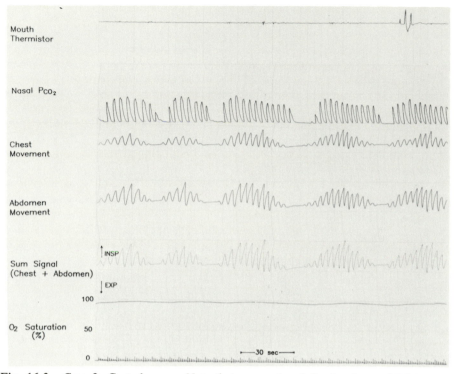

Fig. 16-3. Case 2. Central apnea. Note that apneas (no deflection in nasal PCO_2) are accompanied by total absence of movement in both chest and abdomen channels of inductance plethysmograph (and therefore also in sum signal). The patient was in stage II sleep.

or nasal CO_2 channels) with no movement in the chest or abdomen channels. This establishes these apneas as central. At other times, the patient showed obstructive apneas. However, 80 percent of the apneas were central. REM sleep was associated with central apneas, lasting up to 65 seconds and severe arterial O_2 desaturation.

Tracheostomy with use of a ventilator at night was recommended, and produced improvement in the patient's hypersomnolence and in his daytime arterial PCO_2.

References

1. Phillipson E. Control of breathing during sleep. Am Rev Resp Dis 118:909, 1978
2. Rechtshaffen A, Kales A. A manual of standardized terminology, techniques, and scoring for sleep stages of human subjects. Nat Inst of Health Pub #204, Washington, DC, 1968
3. Bulow K. Respiration and wakefulness in man. Acta Physiol Scand 59:(suppl) 209:1–110, 1963

4. Robin E, Whaley R, Crump C, et al. Alveolar gas tension, pulmonary ventilation and blood pH during physiologic sleep in normal subjects. J Clin Invest 37:981–989, 1958

5. Goethe B, Altose M, Cherniack N. Effect of quiet sleep on resting and CO2 stimulated breathing in humans. J Appl Physiol 50:724–730, 1981

6. Brebbia DR, Altshuler KZ. Oxygen consumption rate and electroencephalographic stage of sleep. Science 150:1621–1623, 1965

7. Snyder F, Hobson JA, Morrison DF, et al. Changes in respiration, heart rate, and systolic blood pressure in human sleep. J Appl Physiol 19:417, 1964

8. Dement W, Kleitman N. Cyclic variation in EEG during sleep and their relation to eye movements, body motility, and dreaming. Electroencephalogr Clin Neurophysiol 9:673, 1957

9. Phillipson E, Kozar L, Rebuch A, et al. Ventilatory and waking responses to CO_2 in sleeping dogs. Am Rev Resp Dis 115:251, 1977

10. Neubaur J, Santiago T, Edelman N. Hypoxic arousal in sleeping cats. Am Rev Resp Dis 121:383A, 1980

12. Sullivan CE, Murphy E, Kozar LF, et al. Waking and ventilatory responses to laryngeal stimulation in sleeping dogs. J Appl Physiol 45:681, 1978

13. Issa FG, Sullivan CE. Arousal and breathing responses to airway occlusion in healthy sleeping adults. J Appl Physiol 55:1113, 1983

14. Strohl K. Upper airway muscles of respiration. Am Rev Resp Dis 124:211–213, 1981

15. Brouillette R, Thach B. A neuromuscular mechanism maintaining extrathoracic airway patency. J Appl Physiol 46:772–779, 1979

16. Sauerland E, Harper R. The human tongue during sleep:electromyographic activity of the genioglossus muscle. Exp Neurol 51:160–170, 1976

17. Duron B. Postural and ventilatory functions of intercostal muscles. Acta Neurobiol Exp 33:355, 1973

18. Strohl K, Hensley M, Hallett M, et al. Activation of upper airway muscles before onset of inspiration in normal humans. J Appl Physiol 49:638–642, 1980

19. Remmers J, deGroot W, Sauerland E, et al. Pathogenesis of upper airway occlusion during sleep. J Appl Physiol 44:931–938, 1978

20. Goldman M, Mead J. Mechanical interaction between the diaphragm and rib cage. J Appl Physiol 35:197, 1973

21. Orem J, Netick A, Dement N. Increased upper airway resistance to rebreathing during sleep in the cat. Electroenceph Clin Neuro 43:14–22, 1977

22. Sleep Disorders Classification Committee, Association of Sleep Disorders Center. Diagnostic classification of sleep and arousal disorders. Sleep 2:21, 1979

23. Guilleminault C, Tilkian A, Dement WC. The sleep apnea syndromes. Ann Rev Med 31:465, 1976

24. Skatrud J, Iber C, Ewart R, et al. Disordered breathing in hypothyroidism. Am Rev Resp Dis 124:325, 1981

25. Guilleminault C, van den Hoed J, Mitler M. Clinical overview of sleep apnea syndromes. In Guilleminault C, Dement WC, (Eds), Sleep Apnea Syndromes. NY, Alan R. Liss, Inc, 1978

26. Orr WC, Martin RJ. Obstructive sleep apnea associated with tonsilar hypertrophy in adults. Arch Int Med 141:990, 1981

27. Conway WA, Bowers GC, Barnes M. Hypersomnolence of intermittent upper airway obstruction: occurrence caused by micrognathia. J Am Med Assoc 237:2740, 1977

28. Coccagnia G, diDonato G, Verucchi P, et al. Hypersomnia with periodic apneas in acquired micrognathia. Arch Neurol 33:769, 1976

29. Olsen K, Sh KW, Staats BA. Surgically correctable causes of sleep apnea syndrome. Otolaryngol Head and Neck Surg 89:726, 1981

30. Guilleminault C, Eldridge FL, Simon FB, et al. Sleep apnea in eight children. Pediatrics 58:23, 1976

31. Guilleminault C, Dement WC. 235 cases of excessive daytime sleepiness. J Neurol Sci 31:13, 1977

32. Lugaresi E, Coccagna G, Farnetti P, et al. Snoring. Electroencephal Clin Neurophys 39:59, 1975

33. Tilkian AG, Guilleminault C, Schroeder JS, et al. Sleep induced apnea syndromes: Prevalence of cardiac arrhythmias and their reversal after tracheostomy. Am J Med 63:348, 1977

34. Tilkian AG, Guilleminault C, Schroeder JS, et al. Hemodynamics in sleep induced apnea. Ann Int Med 85:714, 1976

35. Garay SM, Rapoport DM, Srkin B, et al. Regulation of ventilation in the obstructive sleep apnea syndrome. Am Rev Resp Dis 124:451, 1981

36. Motta J, Guilleminault C, Schroeder JS, et al. Tracheostomy and hemodynamics in sleep induced apnea. Ann Int Med 89:454, 1978

37. Krieger AJ. Sleep apnea produced by cervical cordotomy and other neurosurgical lesions in man, in Guilleminault C, Dement WC (Eds), Sleep Apnea Syndromes. New York, Alan R. Liss, Inc., 1976

38. Severinghaus JW, Mitchell RA. Ondine's curse-failure of respiratory center automaticity while awake. Clin Res 10:122, 1962

39. Plum F, Swanson AG. Abnormalities in central regulation of respiration in acute and convalescent poliomyelitis. Arch Neurol Psych 80:267, 1958

40. Solliday NH, Gaensler EA, Schwaber JR, et al. Impaired central chemoreceptor function and chronic hypoventilation many years following poliomyelitis. Respiration 31:177, 1974

41. Guilleminault C. Sleep apnea syndromes. Impact of sleep and sleep states. Sleep 3:227, 1980

42. Mellins RB, Balfour HH, Turino GM, et al. Failure of automatic control of ventilation (Ondine's curse). Medicine 49:487, 1970

43. Muspratt S. A simple pneumotachograph for qualitative monitoring of respiration and detection of apnea. Am Rev Resp Dis 12:560, 1981

44. Chadha TS, Watson H, Birch S, et al. Validation of respiratory inductive plethysmography using different calibration procedures. Am Rev Respir Dis 125:644–649, 1982

INDEX